D1258178

WILLIAM F. MAAG LIBRARY
YOUNGSTOWN STATE UNIVERSITY

Windsor Bath Library

WILLIAM F. MAAG LIBRARY
YOUNGSTOWN STATE UNIVERSITY

Taping Techniques
Principles and Practice

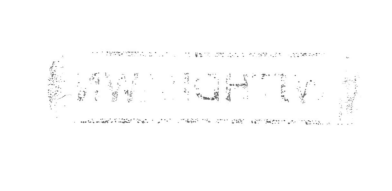

ApbK
538
Black

Taping Techniques:

Principles and Practice

Edited by

Rose Macdonald BA, MCSP, MCPA, SRP
Director, Sports Injury Centre, Crystal Palace National Sports Centre, London, UK

With International Contributors

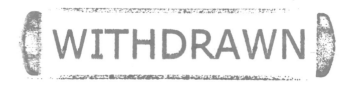
WITHDRAWN

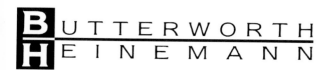
BUTTERWORTH
HEINEMANN

WILLIAM F. MAAG LIBRARY
YOUNGSTOWN STATE UNIVERSITY

Butterworth-Heinemann Ltd
Linacre House, Jordan Hill, Oxford OX2 8DP

A member of the Reed Elsevier group

OXFORD   LONDON   BOSTON
MUNICH   NEW DELHI   SINGAPORE   SYDNEY
TOKYO   TORONTO   WELLINGTON

First published 1994

© Butterworth-Heinemann Ltd 1994

All rights reserved. No part of this publication
may be reproduced in any material form (including
photocopying or storing in any medium by electronic
means and whether or not transiently or incidentally
to some other use of this publication) without the
written permission of the copyright holder except in
accordance with the provisions of the Copyright,
Designs and Patents Act 1988 or under the terms of a
licence issued by the Copyright Licensing Agency Ltd,
90 Tottenham Court Road, London, England W1P 9HE.
Applications for the copyright holder's written permission
to reproduce any part of this publication should be addressed
to the publishers

British Library Cataloguing in Publication Data
Taping Techniques: Principles and Practice
 I. Macdonald, Rose
 617.1

ISBN 0 7506 0577 4

Library of Congress Cataloguing in Publication Data
Taping techniques : principles and practice / edited by Rose
 Macdonald, with international contributors.
 p.   cm.
 Includes bibliographical references and index.
 ISBN 0 7506 0577 4
 1. Bandages and bandaging.   2. Sports—Accidents and
 injuries—Treatment.   3. Sports—Accidents and injuries—
 Prevention.
 I. Macdonald, Rose.
 RD113.T37   1993   93–31803
 617.1'7—dc20   CIP

Composition by Scribe Design, Gillingham, Kent
Printed and bound in Great Britain by The Bath Press, Avon

RD
113
.T37

1994

Contents

Contributors

Chuck Armstrong DipPT, BA(PE), DPT, BEd, MEd, MScPT

Chuck Armstrong worked from 1974 until 1986 as Head Trainer and Physical Therapist at the College of Physical Education at the University of Saskatchewan, Saskatoon. He was Chairman of the Sports Physiotherapy Division of the Canadian Physical Therapy Association between 1981 and 1983. He has been President of the Sport Medicine Council of Canada between 1990 and 1992 and is currently the President of the Sport Medicine Council of Saskatchewan. He has been the Chief Physical Therapist for Athletics Canada since 1976 and has attended six Olympic Games as a Physical Therapist.

Dwayne Dixon

The Late Dwayne 'spike' Dixon was, amongst other things, Instructor of Athletic Training Methods at Indiana University Health, Physical Education and Recreation School from 1950 to 1972. He was a Charter Member of the National Athetic Trainers Association and Past National Director District & National Athetic Trainers Association. He was the first to use ice therapy (cryotherapy) in 1952 and was the author of *Dixonary of Athletic Training*. He entered the Helms Athletic Foundation Hall of Fame in 1970 for noteworthy achievement in Athletic Training.

Garry P. Lapenskie BSc(PE), BSc(PT), MA(PE)

Garry Lapenskie, a practising physiotherapist, has been assigned to medical teams for the 1979 Pan-American Games, 1984 Winter Olympics, 1988 Summer Olympics and the 1990 Commonwealth Games. He is a past Chairman of the Sports Physiotherapy Division of the Canadian Physiotherapy Association and is currently Chairman of the Orthopaedics Division, and Lecturer at the Faculty of Kinesiology at he University of Western Ontario, Canada.

Sue Lennox MCSP, SRP, GradDip Phys

Sue Lennox has worked in Sports Medicine for the past 12 years and was physiotherapist to the Amateur Boxing Association for 3 years. She is a physiotherapist for the Amateur Athletic Association. Previous positions include Deputy Superintendent Physiotherapist at the Crystal Palace Sports Injury Centre and Physiotherapy Manager of the Gordon Sports Medicine Centre, Aberdeen. She has set up sports injury clinics in the public and private sectors.

Rose Macdonald BA, MCSP, MCPA, SRP

Rose Macdonald is the Director of the Sports Injury Centre at Crystal Palace National Sports Centre, London, UK. She is a graduate of the University of Western Ontario, Canada and her physiotherapy training is from Guy's Hospital, London. She has over 15 years experience in Sports Medicine/Physiotherapy and has been actively involved with British Athletics teams at National, International and Olympic competitions for the past 12 years. She lectures widely at home and overseas in Sports Physiotherapy, Injury Prevention and Health. She serves on several National and International Committees relating to Sports Medicine: International Federation of Sports Medicine (Liason Commission), British Association of Sport and Medicine (Executive Committee), and National Sports Medicine Institute of the UK (Board Member), and is Chairman of the Association of Chartered Physiotherapists in Sports Medicine (UK).

Peter Madigan BEd, DPodM, MChS
Peter Madigan is a Podiatrist at the Sports Medicine Centre, Kelvin Hall International Arena, Glasgow and is a Member of the Medical Committee of the Great Scottish Run. He is also a Lecturer in Podiatry at Glasgow Caledonian University.

Sue Nickson BSc, FPodA, DPodM, MChS, SRCh, MBES
Sue Nickson was an executive committee member for the British Association of Sport and Medicine during the 1980s. On various sub-committees for the Yorkshire and Humberside Region of the Sports Council. Sports Podiatrist to various athletic events including the London Marathon. Private practice in Sports Podiatry for many years. Fellow of the Podiatry Association and Past Education Chairman. Initiatior and Member of the Course Development Team for the Post Registration Certificate in Sports Podiatry and the Masters Programme in Sports and Therapy run at the Crewe and Alsager Faculty of the Manchester Metropolitan University. Member of the Society of Chiropodists and Past Member of Council. Chairperson of the Birmingham and District Branch of the Society of Chiropodists. Founder member and past Chairperson of the Manchester Post Graduate Group and the East Pennines Podiatry Group. Member of various branches of the British Association of Sport and Medicine. Member of the International Society of Prosthetists and Orthotists U.K. Member of the Biological Engineering Society.

Jeffrey T. O'Neil M.S., A.T.,C.
Jeff O'Neill is currently Head Athletic Trainer with the Barcelona Dragons Professional Football Club and has been since the league's inception in 1990. Prior to this he was Head Athletic Trainer for Florida Southern College.

Dale Reese BS
Dale Reese is Chief Executive Officer of MCB, Medicinskt Center Billingen, Sweden. He is past President of the Soccer Sports Therapist Association and is a member of the Swedish Sports Medicine Association. He was Head Sport Therapist for the Swedish soccer squad at the 1990 World Cup.

Olivier Rouillon
Olivier Rouillon is Editor of Sport Med. He is also a physiotherapist, and is ex-physician to the national French basket-ball squad. He is a member of the National Medical Commission of the French Basket-ball Federation.

Cathy Stretton OBE, RGN, RCNT, DNCert
Following nurse training at King's College Hospital, London, Cathy Stretton developed a particular interest in Trauma and Emergency Care. She is involved in nurse education at all levels. Formerly visiting lecturer in Clinical Nursing at the University of the South Bank and lecturer in In-Flight Care at the Institute of Advanced Education, Royal College of Nursing. She is currently Director of St John Ambulance, London, developing first-aid training material and programmes, and offering training to Industry and the general public. She is involved in the planning, provision and delivery of first-aid care at major public events in London such as pop concerts, demonstrations, football and all sporting events, especially the London Marathon since its inception.

Kenneth Wright DA, ATC
Ken Wright is Director of Athletic Training Education, The University of Alabama. Prior to that he served as Head Athletic Trainer at the University of North Carolina – Charlotte and Morehead State University. Ken has actively been involved with the US Olympic Committee at both international and national competitions since 1984. Currently he works as a drug crew chief in the USOC drug testing program.

Preface

Functional taping is now acknowledged internationally as having a place in sports medicine. This technique is practised by those involved with caring for the injured. It is widely used during the treatment and rehabilitation programme of the injured in order to aid the healing process by supporting and protecting the injured structures. Functional taping thus allows earlier resumption of activity and the patient is confident in the knowledge that the tissues are supported and protected against reinjury. Sports medicine leans towards early mobilization through functional therapy, and total immobilization in plaster casts is less common. Removable cast bracing is used to enable therapy to continue throughout the postoperative phase. Tape becomes a flexible cast which aids in the prevention of athletic injuries and rests injured parts in order to aid healing. Flexible tape casts limit motion and may be used in many sports where rigid supports are not allowed.

Taping reduces the need for prolonged treatment and reduces time off sport/work for the patient. Many techniques are useful for the non-sports player and may be used by the general practitioner in general practice or in the hospital environment.

My first taping book, *Taping/Strapping: A Practical Guide*, published by BDF Medical in 1985, has been instrumental in keeping me busy tutoring on taping courses throughout the country. The inevitable question asked is, 'When will advanced courses be offered?' Since taping is essentially practical, new techniques are constantly being developed not only to prevent injuries but also to allow patients to return to work/sport more quickly by using tape effectively. Once the basic techniques are mastered, it is then up to the practitioners to modify, change and develop new techniques themselves, always adhering to the basic principles of taping. To aid in the development of new techniques, this book is full of new ideas, which may be used as indicated or modified to suit the situation. The book brings an abundance of international techniques to the reader. The contributors are specialists in their own field and have developed functional taping techniques for various injuries or biomechanical problems.

Podiatry is playing a greater role in sports medicine now. Therefore, there is a contribution on podiatric techniques.

Some 'quickies' or 'many uses' for a strip of tape are also included. Common sense and an imaginative mind can create a simple temporary support. Bandaging now seems to be a thing of the past and is not taught to undergraduate physiotherapy or nursing students. Therefore, a short section on spica bandaging is included. On some occasions a bandage is more appropriate than tape. Spicas are mainly used to hold protective pads/devices in place during training or competition.

Finally, a section on first aid is included for quick reference.

Acknowledgements

I wish to thank all the contributors for sharing their proven techniques with us.

I would also like to thank Butterworth-Heinemann for inviting me to edit the book, for their help in collecting material and for finally producing the book.

I would also like to thank Beiersdorf for their support and Tim Brown, editorial assistant, for his infinite patience in the collection and gathering together of the papers.

Nora Mortimer, graphic designer, must be commended for producing such excellent clear illustrations from a plethora of hand-drawn cartoons – the only way to describe some of the drawings.

Thanks to Diane Scales for allowing me to use the heel bruise technique from her late father's book, *The Dictionary of Athletic Training* by Dwayne 'Spike' Dixon.

I would like to thank my colleague, Barbara Marsden, for helping me to collate the techniques for the book.

Many thanks to St John Ambulance for allowing us to use their illustrations for Figures 14.1–14.6, and to Beiersdorf for giving us their permission to use material from the book *Taping/Strapping: A Practical Guide* (BDF Medical, 1985) for Figures 5.8–5.17, 6.5–6.9, 7.15–7.23, 8.4–8.10, 11.5–11.7 and 11.23.

International terms and definitions

Tensors	Elastic bandage/wrap, non-adhesive
Cohesive	Rubberized bandage which sticks to itself, but not to the skin
Linen tape	Ankle tape – white tape/T tape/porous tape/rigid tape
Skin lube	Lubricant/petroleum jelly
Tufskin	Adhesive/benzoin spray; to anchor tape, underwrap or elastic wrap, reducing blister-causing friction
Cloth wrap	Close-weave cotton material, e.g. triangular bandage or 3.75 cm cloth bandage
Butterfly, hourglass	Fan shapes constructed from tape, used for check rein
Moleskin tape	Soft thick-napped cotton-back cloth
Skin prep	Provides a barrier between the adhesive and surface of the skin – reduces trauma on tape removal
Bed	Bench, couch, plinth

Metric equivalents

½ in	1.25 cm		3 in	7.5/8 cm
1 in	2.5 cm		4 in	10 cm
1.5 in	3.75/3.8/4 cm		6 in	15 cm
2 in	5/6 cm			

Part One

Chapter One

Introduction

R. Macdonald

Taping may be defined as the application of adhesive tape–elastic (stretch) or non-elastic (rigid)–in order to provide support and protection to soft tissues and joints and to minimize swelling and pain after injury.

The application of tape is easy, but if it is not carried out correctly it will be of little value and may even be detrimental. Therefore a knowledge of the basic principles and practical aspects is essential if the full value of the technique is to be attained. Tape should reinforce the normal supportive structures in their relaxed position and protect injured tissues from further damage. Remember when taping a musculotendinous structure in order to reduce stretch–the tape will not protect against the strain inherent in muscular contraction.

Many different techniques are used for injury prevention, treatment, rehabilitation and proprioception. Various techniques are illustrated in this manual together with different philosophies expressed by the contributors – many of whom are eminent physical therapists in their respective countries.

Initial use

Initially tape is applied to protect the injured structure, during the treatment and rehabilitation programme:

- to hold dressings and pads in place
- to compress recent injury, thus reducing bleeding and swelling

- to protect from further injury by supporting ligaments, tendons and muscles
- to limit unwanted joint movement
- to allow healing without stressing the injured structures
- to protect and support the injured structure in a functional position during the exercise, strengthening and proprioceptive programme

It must be clearly understood that taping is not a substitute for treatment and rehabilitation, but is an adjunct to the total injury care programme.

Return to activity

On return to activity the injured area is still at risk, therefore reinjury can be prevented by taping the weakened area, with the aim of restricting joint and muscle movement to within safe limits. This allows performance with confidence.

Laxity of joints and hypermobility may also be supported with adhesive tape in order to reduce the risk of injury during sport.

Taping principles

A thorough assessment is necessary before taping any structure. Know the answers to the following before commencing:

- How did the injury occur?
- Has the injury been thoroughly assessed?
- Are your familiar with the anatomy and biomechanics of the parts involved?
- What structures were damaged?
- What tissues need protection and support?
- What movements must be restricted?
- Is complete immobilization necessary at this stage?
- Are you familiar with the technique?
- Do you have suitable materials for the taping techniques?
- Can you visualize the purpose for which the tape is being applied?

Note: Should you consider applying tape to a player, ensure that the use of tape does not contravene the rules of the sport, thus making the player ineligible to participate.

Taping guidelines

Prepare the area to be taped. Wash, dry and shave the skin in a downward direction. Remove oils for better adhesion. Cover broken lesions before taping; an electric shaver avoids cutting the skin. Check if the athlete is allergic to tape, spray etc. Apply lubricated protective padding to friction and pressure areas. Apply adhesive spray for skin protection and better tape adhesion. Apply underwrap for sensitive skin. If the area is frequently taped, move the anchor point on successive tapings to prevent skin irritation and infection.

Tape application

Apply tape only to skin which is at room temperature. Have all the required materials at hand. Have the athlete and yourself in a position which will cause minimal fatigue, e.g. the couch should be at an appropriate height, etc. Place the joint in a functional position, with minimum stress on the injured structure. Ensure that the ligaments are in their short-ened position. Use the correct type, width and amount of tape for the job in hand and apply strips of tape in sequential order, the first strips applied vertical to the injured soft tissue or structure. Overlap successive strips by half. Lay each strip with a particular purpose in mind,

pulling a small amount from the roll at a time. Apply tape smoothly and firmly, gradually angled, and 'flow' with the shape of the limb.

The tape should conform with even pressure and must be effective and comfortable. For difficult acute-angled areas, rip the end of the tape longitudinally into strips–small strips are easier to conform by lapping them over each other. Tape applied directly to the skin gives maximum support.

Avoid:
- excessive traction on skin, as it may lead to skin breakdown
- gaps and wrinkles–these may cause blisters, therefore overlap each strip by half
- continuous circumferential strips–single strips are more likely to produce a uniform pressure
- excessive layers of tape, too tight an application and using rigid tape around muscles–this may impair circulation and neural transmission.

- Explain the function of the tape to the athlete and how it should feel. On completion, check that the technique is functional and comfortable

Tape removal

Leaving tape on for too long a period may lead to skin breakdown. Tape should not be left on for more than 24 hours. Remove tape carefully–peel it back on itself, watching the skin for breakdown. Push the skin away from the tape while pulling the tape along the axis of the limb.

Never rip tape off, especially from the plantar aspect of the foot. Use a tape cutter or bandage scissors for safe, fast removal. Lubricate the tip with petroleum jelly and slide it parallel to the skin in the natural soft tissue channels.

Check the skin for damage–apply lotion to restore skin moisture. Check if there was adequate stability and control. Are any changes necessary next time?

Taping terms

Anchors The first strips of tape to be applied above and below the injury site and to which subsequent strips are attached. Anchors minimize traction on the skin, and are applied without tension.

Support strips, stirrups To restrict unwanted sideways movement.

Gibney/horizontal strips To add stability to the joint. *Note:* When stirrups and Gibney strips are used alternately, they form a basketweave pattern.

Reinforcing strips Adhesive strips to restrict movement and add tensile strength to strategic areas when applied over stretch tape.

Check reins To restrict range of motion during activity.

Lock strips To secure the cut end of stretch tape, which tends to roll back on itself. Secure check reins in place. Neatly finish the tape job when applied over anchors (fill strips).

Heel locks To give additional support to the subtalar and ankle joints.

Taping and wrapping products

Good-quality tape should adhere readily and maintain adhesion despite perspiration and activity.

Non-stretch adhesive tape has a non-yielding cloth backing and is used for the following:

- to support inert structures, e.g. ligaments, joint capsule
- to limit joint movement
- to protect against re-injury
- to secure ends of stretch tape
- to reinforce stretch tape

Non-stretch tape should be torn by hand to maintain tension during application. It is important to be able to tear the tape from various positions–practice will help to attain a high level of efficiency. *Technique.* Tear the tape close to the roll, keeping it taut. Hold the tape with the thumb and index fingers close together. Rip the tape quickly in scissors fashion. Practice tearing a strip of tape into very small pieces.

Stretch (elastic) adhesive tape conforms to the contours of the body, allowing for normal tissue expansion and is used for the following:

- to compress and support soft tissue, e.g. muscle
- to provide anchors for muscle when it is applied on to the skin without tension

When applying *stretch* adhesive tape, allow the last 2 cm to recoil before sticking down. Stretch tape will not give mechanical support to ligaments. Heavy-duty stretch adhesive tape cannot be torn by hand and must be cut with scissors; some light stretch tape may be torn by hand.

Stretch adhesive tape is available with:

- one-way stretch–in length or width
- two-way stretch–in length and width

Hypoallergenic adhesive non-stretch and stretch tapes are available, offering an alternative to conventional zinc oxide adhesive mass. Both non-stretch and stretch tapes can be obtained with water-repellent properties.

Storage

Tape with zinc oxide adhesive mass is susceptible to temperature change and should be stored in a cool place. Tape should be left in its original packing until required. Partially used rolls should be put in an air-tight container (e.g. cooler box or plastic box) and not left on shelves. At temperatures over 20°C the adhesive mass becomes very sticky, making the unwind tension much stronger and consequently more difficult to work with. Non-stretch tape is also more difficult to tear when warm. Tapes with hypoallergenic adhesive mass are not susceptible to temperature change.

Taping products

Underwrap/prowrap A thin polyurethane foam material used to protect sensitive skin from zinc oxide adhesive mass.

Gauze squares Foam squares, 'heel and lace pads', are used to protect areas susceptible to stress and friction.

Padding Felt, foam rubber or other materials for protecting sensitive areas.

Adhesive spray Applied to make skin tacky and thus help underwrap, protective pads, or tape adhere to the skin more readily.

Petroleum jelly Applied to protective pads to lubricate areas of stress and so reduce friction and irritation to the tissues.

Talcum powder Used to remove adhesive residue where necessary; it also prevents stretch tape from rolling at the edges.

Cohesive bandage Adheres to itself but not to the skin and can be used for light compression or applied over tape to prevent unravelling in water.

Tubular bandage Can be applied over completed tape job to help set the tape.

Tape cutter Allows quick and safe removal of tape.

Bandage scissors Flat-ended scissors for safe removal of tape.

Dehesive spray Breaks down the adhesive mass and allows tape to be removed easily

Tape remover Available as spray, solution or wipes to clean adhesive residue from the skin.

Elastic bandage/tensor Used for compression and for traditional spicas.

Cloth wrap Used for ankle wraps, triangular bandages, collar and cuff support.

Chapter Two

The history of taping

D. Reese

There is evidence that points towards the use of different glue masses, together with the application of cloth of some type of outer covering, since the beginning of recorded history. From later ancient cultures there have been many examples of the use of tape or at least sticky masses that had some type of healing effect and that were applied directly to the skin for local injuries. One is aware that for this purpose the ancient Greeks used a mixture of olive oil, lead oxide and water. Indeed, this very mixture became popular because reportedly it had a soothing and healing effect for a variety of complaints.

The Greek recipe stood more or less unchanged until modern history added resins and beeswax, and the mass became known as *emplastrum resinae*. In the middle of the 18th century an important additive, Indian rubber, became available and, when added to the mixture, made the glue much better by increasing the tackiness, and making both application and removal from the skin easier (unnamed authors, 1972).

Towards the end of the 19th century zinc oxide (in collaboration with researchers) was added. This reduced the amount of skin irritation caused by tape and increased the number of indications for tape in the medical profession. Later refinements in the backing which have more specific applications to different indications, combined with attempts to make the tape lighter, water-resistant and to give better skin acceptability, have made tape a common component of the medical profession.

More recently, modern technology and awareness of the different components in a tape that can cause skin irritation have led to the development of acrylics and synthetic elastomers that virtually eliminate skin irritation and increase the time a person can be in contact with tape; this further enhances the indications for use of tape.

Tape has been in use to support joints and prevent injuries in athletics since the beginning of this century (Glimstaed, 1980). In the USA different techniques have become standard in sports on high school, collegiate and professional levels; indeed, some make the use of preventive taping of the ankle mandatory for participation.

This chapter will take a closer look at the more orthopaedic use of taping techniques, in particular those techniques used within sports to prevent an injury occurring, or to protect soft tissue from further injury during the healing and hardening phase after injury, during active rehabilitation, or indeed even during participation. The basic idea of tape use in sports and rehabilitation is described as follows: tape should support a weakened part of the body by means of preventing the motion in the body part that can cause further insult to the weakened body part without the taping technique compromising the biomechanical function of the body as a whole (Andréasson and Edberg, 1983). This leads us to the view that tape has three distinct usages and techniques within sports, depending on the desired function and the amount of force that will be applied to the body part:

WILLIAM F. MAAG LIBRARY
YOUNGSTOWN STATE UNIVERSITY

1. for acute injuries
2. for prevention of further insult to the body part
3. for rehabilitational purposes, giving support and guidance

In other words, tape is used to prevent the soft tissues from becoming further injured or ruptured and at the same time allows an acceptable range of motions so that normal everyday activity can be maintained. It is important to realize that tape is applied directly to the skin in most cases to support underlying structural soft tissue such as ligaments and joint capsules. Taping of muscle strains and tears is hard to understand since a tape applied to the skin cannot prevent the ruptured ends from separating during work (Andréasson *et al.*, 1980). The skin can be displaced against underlying tissue in most places, especially over the extremities. Mechanically speaking, the effect of tape over areas where this displacement is relatively large is highly doubtful (Andréasson *et al.*, 1980; Andréasson and Edberg, 1983). Taping methods used in sports have one thing in common–that the best supportive results are achieved over joints and body parts where the skin's mobility can be locked or restricted in one or more directions.

How does one tape?

Since the aims of taping and sites of a taped body part differ, it is difficult to give any general rules to follow that will apply wherever tape is applied. However the general principle of taping is rather constant and can be illustrated in the following manner.

Anchors are applied either circularly or semicircularly to either side of the injured area

both to strengthen and to reduce the elasticity of the skin. Supportive strips of varying degrees of viscoelasticity and direction of maximal energy uptake are applied between the anchors in accordance with the desired support and function to be maintained (Figure 2.1).

If one is taping with the intent of giving biomechanical support over a joint, then taking away a lot of the elasticity of the skin is necessary; this can be most easily achieved around the feet, hands, fingers and wrist. However, if the taping is applied to remind the patient of a movement that can further aggravate the injury, then one is making use of the skin's proprioceptors to create a simulated pain reflex. The afferent nerves of the skin send signals and cause an efferent response in avoidance of the afferent stimulation (Millar, 1973; Karlsson *et al.*, 1985). One could use the analogy of the tape working as an amplifier in a stereo system to enhance the sound.

Technological textile studies have shown that rigid tape, the type most often used in sports, is not as strong as the ligaments it is meant to support (Andréasson *et al.*, 1980). However there are studies that show that taping of the ankle, for example, does reduce the amount of injuries (Garrick and Requa, 1973; Lindenberger *et al.*, 1985). This contradiction between the clinical and mechanical properties of tape has suggested that tape has two functions: one is supporting and decreasing the passive instability of a joint and the other is enhancing the active stability. This is achieved by skin receptors facilitating signals from the intramuscular and joint receptors (Mayhew, 1972; Furnich *et al.*, 1980; Andréasson *et al.*, 1985). Functional instability, which is the subjective summary of a patient's complaints about the joint, can be divided into several possible causes–mechanical instability, muscle weakness, proprioceptive deficit, deafferentation of the joint and motor incoordination (Freeman, 1965; Freeman *et al.*, 1965; Tropp *et al.*, 1985). The proprioceptive deficit and the deafferentation of the joint, muscle weakness and motor coordination can be regained after an injury in most cases through re-education, such as a balance board and physical therapy. Tape used as part of the rehabilitation and prevention of further insult to a joint may theoretically increase this process. Electromyogram studies on the muscle protecting the ankle from lateral ankle sprains showed no

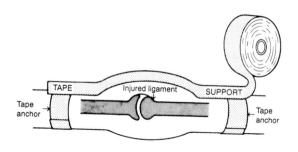

Figure 2.1

difference in the response time between a healthy untaped ankle and a healthy taped ankle, but did show a significant increase in unhealthy taped ankles, supporting the hypothesis that tape can enhance the active stability around a joint (Karlsson *et al.*, 1985). Further studies are necessary but the tendency is established, and the results are dependent on the biomechanical configuration of the joint and the physiological status, combined with the mobility of the skin.

When a taped person is active the body part bends, stretches, twists, turns and compresses. This means that the tape is following the same movement. In order to get the best effect of tape it is necessary to look at different factors that can affect the final results, such as tensile strength, skin, sweat retention, practice, technique and observation. When applying tape, tensile strength is usually placed with a certain pretension, which in turn means that a strain is placed on the tape from the very beginning, producing a loss of part of the strength of the tape. This loss of strength will increase in time with repeated tensions from activity. The resultant elongation is correlated to the number of threads in the backing in both directions–the more, the better. As for the skin, because the anchors and part of the supports are placed directly on the skin, the proprioreceptors in the skin are utilized. This means that we become aware through reflexes that a certain range of motion should be avoided and a muscle response is accordingly activated. This places great demands on the type of adhesive used. Because of increased body temperature and friction the viscosity of the glue should not become fluid, thus leaving the backing and decreasing the contact with the skin. The adhesive should also be porous to allow sweat, which is of high concentration, to be absorbed by a medium of lower concentration such as a sock, or to evaporate so that the contact between the skin and adhesive remains undisturbed. Observation, technique and practice for the different areas of the body to be taped are necessary to optimize the function of tape. It is not until one comprehends how biomechanical corrections and rehabilitative reminders can be achieved by placing a few pieces of tape in an organized fashion that one realizes how amazing taping is. Practice makes perfect.

References

Andréasson G, Edberg B. (1983) Mechanical tape to prevent athletic injuries. *Textile Research Journal*.

Andréasson G, Edberg B, Peterson L, Renström P (1980) Mechanical function analysis of tape (in Swedish). *Läkartidningen* **77**, 33628–3629

Andréasson G, Reese D, Renström P (1985) Subjective experience of medical tape used to prevent athletic ankle injuries. Thesis. Department of Textile Technology, Chalmers University of Technology, Gothenburg, Sweden.

Freeman MAR (1965) Instability of the foot after injuries to the lateral ligament of the ankle. *Journal of Bone and Joint Surgery* **47-B**, 669–677.

Freeman MAR, Dean MRE, Hanham IWF (1965) The etiology of the foot after injuries to the lateral ligament of the ankle. *Journal of Bone and Joint Surgery* **47-B**, 678–685.

Furnich RM, Ellison AE, Guermi GJ (1980) The measured effect of taping on combined foot and ankle motion before and after exercise. *American Journal of Sports Medicine* **9**, 165–170.

Garrick JG, Requa RK (1973) Role of external support in prevention of ankle sprains. *Medical Science of Sports* **5**, 200–203.

Glimstaed OH (1980) *Adhesive Plaster Bandaging in Athletics*, 2nd edn. Johnson & Johnson, USA.

Karlsson J, Andréasson G, Reese D, Peterson L, Renström P (1985) The effect of external ankle support on ankle joint instability–an EMG study. Thesis. Department of Textile Technology, Chalmers University of Technology, Gothenburg, Sweden.

Lindenberger U, Andréasson G, Reese D, Peterson L, Ranström P (1985) The effect of prophylactic taping of ankles. Thesis. Department of Textile Technology, Chalmers University of Technology, Gothenburg, Sweden.

Mayhew JL (1972) Effects of ankle taping on motor performance. *Athletic Training* **7**, 1011.

Millar J (1973) Joint afferent fibres responding to muscle stretch vibration and contraction. *Brain Research* **63**, 380–838.

Tropp H, Ekstrand J, Gillquist J (1985) Pronator muscle weakness in functional instability of the ankle joint.

(1972) *Professional Uses of Adhesive Tape*, 3rd edn. Johnson & Johnson, USA.

Chapter Three

Foot types, mechanics and therapy

S. Nickson and P. Madigan

This chapter aims to summarize the main mechanical problems encountered by the sports participant. Diagnostic clues are listed to facilitate decision-making by the practitioner. A range of quick treatments is given and methods of achieving them. Clinical padding can be effectively combined with a range of tapings and strappings, described elsewhere in this book. Longer-term treatments are also discussed. Further reading is listed at the end of the chapter for those who wish to study the subject further.

Types of first aid padding

Plantar metatarsal pads (PMPs)

Uses
- redistribute load over a larger area
- alter the timing of load over a pressure point
- act as a locator for medication
- reduce friction over the metatarsal head area

Materials of construction

Adhesive
- Chiropodist's felt–semicompressed felt with or without adhesive
- Open-cell, synthetic rubber cushioning (Swanfoam, Molefoam)

Insole and orthotic prescription
- Poron
- PPT
- Spenco

Method of construction (Fig. 3.1)

Outline of full thickness of pad in 5 or 7 mm semicompressed felt. The anterior border may extend over the second, third and fourth metatarsal heads or all five, depending on function.

Bevelling or skiving the borders of the pad will make it adhere better to the skin and prevent the patient feeling an abrupt ridge all round the pad (*Figure 3.2*).

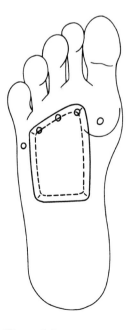

Figure 3.1

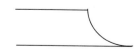

Figure 3.2

Mechanics of the pad and materials used

- Load is more evenly distributed over the surface of the pad rather than being concentrated at the metatarsal heads.
- Load is reduced over a pressure point by making a U-shaped cut-out in the pad. This increases the length of time that surrounding areas are in contact with the ground (and reduces the time for the pressure point).
- Reduces problems from skin friction, which occurs at the foot–shoe interface, by inducing friction to occur between the pad and the shoe.
- If the aim of the pad is to alter loading, then chiropodist's felt should be used. Open-cell, synthetic rubber cushioning will assist in decelerating the forefoot and reducing force immediately before impact.
- They are easily cut to shape and can be adhered to the foot or to the insole of a running shoe. They are, however, short-term first aid materials and, if successful, a similarly shaped insole should be constructed.

Variations on a theme: plantar cover pads

Uses
- cushion the whole metatarsophalangeal joint area (ball of the foot)
- redistribute load over a larger area
- reduce friction over the metatarsal head area
- alter the timing of loading over the area
- act as a locator for medication

Materials of construction

Adhesive or replaceable padding
- Chiropodist's felt
- Open-cell, synthetic rubber cushioning (Swanfoam, Molefoam)

Insole or orthotic prescription
- Poron
- PPT
- Spenco

Method of construction

The pad is the same shape and size as the adhesive version. It may be adhered directly into the shoe, or a template made from thin cardboard or regenerated leather board (Texon) or thin EVA (Evalon) is cut to the shape of the inside of the shoe. The patient wears this in the shoe for at least 1 week, to produce a dynamic imprint of the plantar surface of the foot. From this, the metatarsal heads and centre heel can be identified and used as reference points for the pad. The pad is cut to shape, bevelled and adhered to the insole base and covered with a top cover.

Mechanics of the pad and materials used (comparison of the different materials required)

There is little to choose between the open-cell (Poron, PPT) and the closed-cell (Spenco) orthotic materials in terms of reducing pressure and force under the foot.

The open-cell construction of Poron and PPT is said to channel sweat and moisture away from the surface of the foot, thus keeping it cooler. The closed-cell neoprene rubber, Spenco, contains entrapped bubbles, or cells which are not interconnected, causing it to retain heat and moisture. This may be a consideration with middle- and long-distance events.

Both types of materials are available with a pre-adhered nylon top cover which helps reduce friction.

Shaft pad

Uses
- to realign one metatarsal with the rest, e.g. in Morton's neuroma, apply to third or fourth metatarsal
- with a dorsiflexed first metatarsal and medial cuneiform, to bring the ground to the metatarsal
- to provide protection to a lesion such as a hard corn, overlying the metatarsophalangeal head (a crescent or cavity may be included)
- to provide protection to a lesion such as a hard corn, overlying the plantar surface of the interphalangeal joint of the first toe (big toe)

Materials of construction

Adhesive
- Chiropodist's felt

Insole or orthotic prescription
- Poron
- PPT
- Spenco

Made in the same way as the PMP, and adhered:

1. directly to the insole of the shoe
2. to an insole base

Mechanics

The shaft pad has a similar function to the PMP in that it provides protection to a lesion by increasing the available surface area through which pressure can be dissipated and by altering the timing during which the pressure is applied.

The surface area is, however, very much smaller than that of the PMP but it is a useful form of padding where space within the shoe is at a premium.

D pad or valgus filler pad

There are several variations of this pad.

Uses
- to reduce the effects of foot strain by filling the inner longitudinal arch or lateral longitudinal arch
- to facilitate the effect of an inversion or eversion strapping

Variations

It may be constructed with a PMP to increase effective loading of the foot.

Materials of construction

Adhesive
- Semicompressed felt

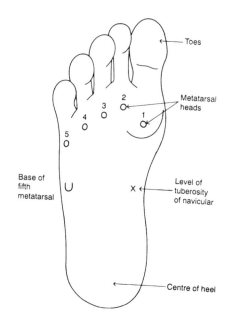

Figure 3.3

Replaceable
- Semicompressed felt on an elastic net webbing or tubular elastic bandage

Insole or orthotic construction
- Poron
- PPT
- Dense Plastazote

Landmarks (Fig. 3.3)

- Toes
- Metatarsal heads
- Base of fifth metatarsal
- Level of tuberosity of navicular
- Centre of heel

There are several shapes described for this type of padding:

1. The full thickness should extend from behind the first metatarsal head, following the curve of the long arch, and finish anterior to the weight-bearing surface or the heel. Some colleagues find that an extension on the medial side extending up to the navicular can be even more effective.

Strapping the pad to the foot can incorporate any of the inversion strappings or plantar tension strappings.

2. The D shape is the other way round, with the straight edge extending from behind/ posterior to the first metatarsophalangeal joint to the anterior aspect of the calcaneum and placed along the midline of the foot.

D pad (Fig. 3.4)

Mechanics

The available room for the foot to pronate is reduced by filling the arch of the foot or its corresponding space in the shoe. Pronation lengthens the foot and, if excessive, may strain structures on the plantar surface. Reducing the degree of pronation will give relative rest and support to the plantar structures.

The pad may also be of benefit in compartment syndromes of the leg where muscles are working excessively to reduce pronation.

Heel pad (Fig. 3.5)

Uses
- Sore heel–plantar surface or posterior surface (from heel tab)
- Achilles tendinitis
- Equinus and overuse syndromes
- Location of medication
- Soft tissue trauma

Materials

Adhesive
- Semicompressed felt
- Sponge rubber
- Open-cell, synthetic rubber cushioning (Swanfoam, Molefoam)

Replaceable
- Tubular bandage incorporating semicompressed felt or sponge rubber
- Silicone rubbers as heel cups (Viscoheel) or incorporated into tubular bandage (Silipos, or self-made from a variety of products)
- Sorbothane preformed heel pad

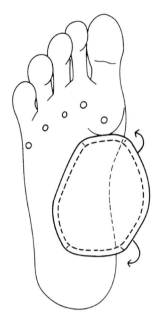

Figure 3.4

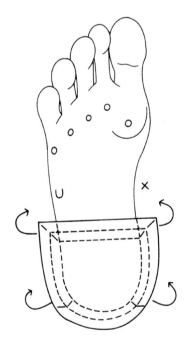

Figure 3.5

Insole or orthotic construction
- Poron
- PPT
- Plastazote
- Sorbothane

Methods of construction (Fig. 3.6)

1. Locate painful area.
2. Cut full thickness of pad to follow margins of the plantar surface of the heel, extending to the anterior weight-bearing border. *Do not* forget to allow some extra material for a bevelled edge, which will make the pad easier to adhere to the foot.
3. If necessary, create a cavity or aperture over the painful area.
4. A combination of felt and sponge rubber can create a cushion effect directly over the painful area, whilst the felt will alter the timing of the loading.

This pad can be incorporated with ankle and arch strapping/taping and Achilles tendon strapping/taping.

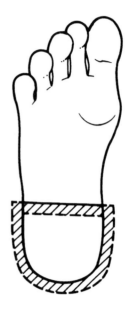

Figure 3.6

Mechanics

For Achilles tendinitis, heel bumps and equinus problems the pad acts by lifting the heel and reducing the degree of dorsiflexion required at the ankle to achieve footflat. A fairly firm material is best and should be placed under the existing insole of the sports shoe.

For plantar heel problems shock attenuation is improved and peak loading reduced with synthetic rubber (Poron, PPT) or viscoelastic (Sorbothane, Viscoheel) material.

Variations

1. Medial/lateral wedge may be incorporated into a heel pad to alter the effects of excessive pronation/supination temporarily.
2. Rose's bar–a rectangular piece of felt cut to conform to the anterior weight-bearing surface of the heel (Fig. 3.7). It has been used to alleviate the effect of plantar fasciitis and works well when incorporated into the specialist strappings for this condition.

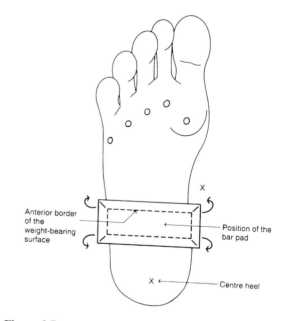

Figure 3.7

Mechanics

The felt bar supports the anterior part of the calcaneum and reduces strain on the plantar fascia during weight-bearing.

Wedges

Uses
- Medial heel wedges (Fig. 3.8) are effective in foot strain and overuse syndromes associated with excessive pronatory forces.

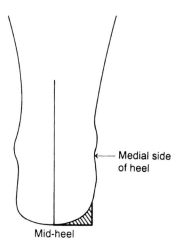

Figure 3.8

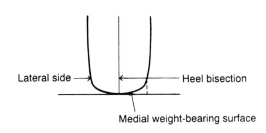

Figure 3.9

Heel wedge

Lateral heel wedges (Fig. 3.9) are effective in cases of repetitive lateral ankle sprains and associated supinatory foot conditions. A lateral flare or flange may be required to overcome the supinatory forces.

Methods of construction

Adhesive
1. Take a piece of felt that is just larger than half the plantar heel area.
2. Bevel away the full thickness to accommodate the mid-heel weight-bearing surface.
3. Adhere to inside of shoe or foot.
4. Incorporate into an inversion or eversion strapping, depending on the result required.

Note: Many sports shoes have removable insoles and wedges can be adhered to the undersurface of these with great effect.

Insole or orthotic construction

If greater control is required than achieved by the aforementioned temporary measures, then an accurate non-weight-bearing foot cast should be taken. The preferred position is in the subtalar joint neutral position and is out of the scope of this book.

Materials

Rigid and semirigid thermoplastics, incorporating wedges constructed from:

● closed-cell rubber
● Poron
● PPT
● EVA

Mechanics

At heel strike the normal foot is in a supinated position. From this position it pronates to decelerate the leg and attenuate shock by unlocking the joints and allowing the bones to become loose and mobile. The foot must quickly halt this pronation and lock the joints, by returning to a supinated position, to become a stable weight-bearing and propulsive platform.

Problems occur when the joints of the foot, for whatever reason, are not in the right place at the right time.

See the section on common foot types, later in this chapter.

Dorsal pads

A range of protective pads can be used to great effect for single or multiple lesions.

Dorsal crescent pad (Fig. 3.10)

Uses
● Protection for a corn, blister, laceration, pressure point
● Vehicle for a medicament
● Relief of shoe pressure

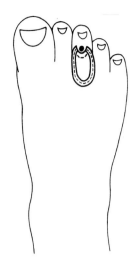

Figure 3.10

Materials

Adhesive
- Semicompressed felt
- Sponge rubber

Replaceable
- Semicompressed felt
- Sponge rubber
- Tubular open-cell foam (polyethylene, e.g. Tubifoam)
- Silipos/silicone orthodigita

Example

Hard corn, etc. on lesser toe which is hammered or clawed.

The full thickness should extend from just posterior to the lesion, down the long axis of the toe, finishing clear of the next articulation.

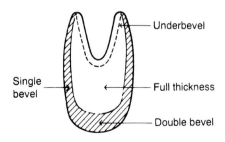

Figure 3.11

An underbevel (Fig. 3.11) protects the lesion and an overbevel blends the pad into the rest of the toe, improving adhesion to the toe.

The medial and lateral borders should match those of the toe. The bevelling extends into the interdigital spaces to improve adhesion, but does not interfere with toe function.

The pad may be held on by a T-shaped strapping or with tubular gauze if a dressing is incorporated into the pad.

Variations

Multiple dorsal crescents can be constructed to protect all or any of the lesser toes (Fig. 3.12).

Note: Avoid limiting extension of the toes and webbing by plantarflexing the toes before adhering pad and strapping.

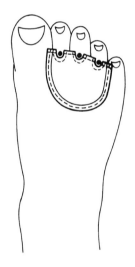

Figure 3.12

Materials

Adhesive and replaceable
- Semicompressed felt: 5 or 7 mm
- Sponge rubber
- Silicones (polydimethylsiloxane)

Method of construction

Ensure a snug fit to each lesion. Measure the required width and depth of pad directly from the foot. Extend the main bulk of the pad proximally, so that the bevelled edge blends with the dorsum of the foot in the area of the metatarsophalangeal joints.

Strap the pad on by using a 2.5 cm hypoallergenic tape halfway across the dorsal aspect of the second toe and taking around the plantar surface of the second toe and up on to the dorsum. *Note*: Do not allow the toes to be totally encircled, nor the tape to become too tight, as this may cause skin and circulatory problems.

Repeat for the fourth toe.

Apply a curved base strap to the proximal edge of the pad, with the toes plantarflexed. This minimizes the drag effect of the dorsal skin.

Silicones

Various proprietary silicone putty compounds are available, either premade into pads contained within a stretch knit material (e.g. Silipos) or with a catalyst for bespoke manufacture.

Digital props/splints (Fig. 3.13)

Uses
● Single- or multiple-clawed, mallet or hammer toes which are flexible: their position needs modification

Materials

Adhesive
● Semicompressed felt

Replaceable
● Semicompressed felt
● Poron
● PPT
● Plastazote
● Silicone

Methods of construction: dorsal

The full thickness of the pad should extend from the distal interphalangeal joint proximally towards the toe web.

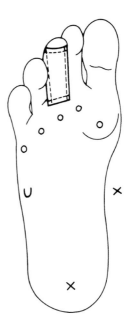

Figure 3.13

The bevel should protect any dorsal lesions. Medial and lateral bevels should extend to the sides of the second and fourth toes for secure adherence. The dorsal prop/splint can be combined with an adhesive plaster prop/splint to increase the effectiveness of both pads.

Mechanics

Digital padding is designed to protect lesions or other areas of pressure by increasing surface area, thereby reducing peak pressure. Some correction of digital alignment can be achieved where the problem is due to soft tissue contracture, but this requires long-term management which is best suited to bespoke silicone orthodigita.

Horseshoe pad (Fig. 3.14)

Uses
● to protect single lesions on very clawed or hammer toes, where minimal movement is available for correction

Materials

Adhesive
● Semicompressed felt

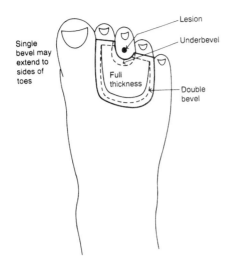

Figure 3.14

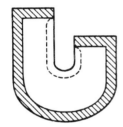

Figure 3.15

Replaceable
● Semicompressed felt
● Poron
● PPT
● Plastazote
● Silicone

Method of manufacture (Fig. 3.15)

This pad is similar to a dorsal crescent but extended medially and laterally to provide bulk and protection on adjacent toes. The bevelling and extent of the pad are also similar.

It may be necessary to provide extra bulk immediately proximal to the lesion. Toe straps can be used as for the dorsal crescent and a base strap will be required to ensure good adhesion.

Replaceable pad

The above procedure is followed, incorporating an elastic net toe loop for ease of use. Reverse the felt and cover the adhesive with tape.

Interdigital pads

Uses
● to prevent mediolateral compression
● to increase interdigital ventilation
● to realign toe relationships

Materials

Adhesive
● Semicompressed felt
● Sponge rubber

Replaceable
● Tubular foam–open-cell
● Silicone orthodigita

Methods

The interdigital wedge is a trapezium-shaped pad, conforming to the dorsoplantar margins of adjacent toes. It extends from the webbing to the distal interphalangeal joint or further if the lesion is located distally.

It is bevelled all the way round and adhered to the toe with flexible strapping to prevent constriction of soft tissue and blood flow.

Mechanics

There is little space available between adjacent toes, particularly those which already show lesions due to mediolateral compression. Care must be taken to make the pad big enough to do the job, but small enough to avoid causing problems between other toes or between the fifth toe and the shoe.

Dumbbell pad (Fig. 3.16)

Uses
● to realign proximal phalanges as they rotate and compress soft tissue on and over the metatarsal head, when a soft corn has been produced.

Method

The full thickness should extend for the total length of the interspace and be as wide as the

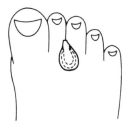

Figure 3.16a

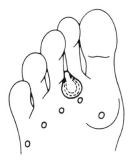

Figure 3.16b

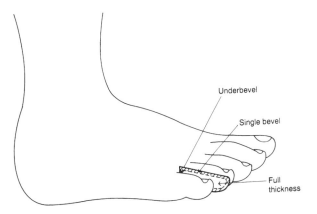

Figure 3.18

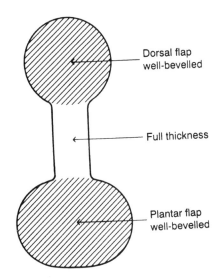

Figure 3.17

interspace. The dorsal and plantar flaps (dumbbells) facilitate pad location and adherence. Tape may be used to increase pad security on both flaps.

Mechanics

The plantar flap raises the metatarsal and its proximal phalanx, while the dorsal flap placed over the adjacent metatarsal pushes it down, ensuring the realignment of the bony prominences which have caused the corn. The section of the pad within the interspace will act as an interdigital wedge.

Replaceable wedges (Fig. 3.18)

These can be constructed from clinical padding but manufacture of a wedge from one of the range of silicone putties is the most effective orthodigita.

Apical pads

Uses
● protection of high-compression/friction areas

Materials

Adhesive
● Semicompressed felt
● Open-cell, synthetic rubber (Swanfoam, Molefoam)
● Sponge rubber

Replaceable
● Commercial apical toe covers in foam
● Commercial silicone devices (e.g. Silipos)
● Bespoke made silicone orthodigita

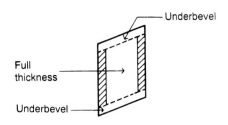

Figure 3.19

Common foot types

Ideal foot relationships when subject is standing (Fig. 3.20)

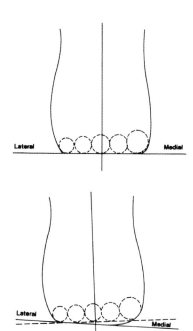

Figure 3.20

Methods

A strip of material is cut to equate to the distance from the dorsal distal interphalangeal joint to the plantar distal interphalangeal joint. The width is just wider than the toe to allow for bevelling.

Note: Care must be taken to protect the nail plate and bed from the long-term effects of adhesive by either:

1. stripping off the adhesive in this area or
2. applying gauze, tape or appropriate material to eliminate the adhesive in this area.

Occasionally it is helpful to create a cavity in the pad directly over the lesion.

Apical crescent

This is a modification of a dorsal crescent pad and is most effective when made as an integral part of a plantar toe prop, otherwise the forces applying to the apex of the toe will still cause the toe to buckle.

Mechanics

The apex of the toe is not designed for weight-bearing and has little fatty padding. If the toe cannot be realigned, an apical pad of felt will increase the surface area over which load is distributed during ground contact and particularly propulsion. A degree of cushioning can be given to the apex with the use of cellular rubbers.

Rearfoot varus

Definition

The neutral position of the subtalar joint is inverted to the long axis of the lower leg, causing the joint to compensate during weight-bearing by pronating to bring the medial side of the foot into ground contact.

Clinical variations

Uncompensated rearfoot varus

Clues to look for:
- Pinch callus on the border of the first and fifth metatarsophalangeal joints
- Spin or rotational callus beneath the fifth metatarsal head
- Lateral heel sprain
- Soft corn or hard corn between fourth and fifth toes

- Tailor's bunion (fifth metatarsophalangeal joint)
- Callus under second and fourth metatarsal heads

Quick treatment
- Medial heel wedge
- PMP

Longer-term treatment
- Biomechanical assessment, gait analysis and orthotic–shoe prescription (refer to a podiatrist); modification to training programme

Partially compensated rearfoot varus

This is where the foot can pronate but not sufficiently to allow full foot-loading in the time sequence.

Clues to look for:
- Haglund's deformity (heel bumps)
- Inverted heel at mid-stance
- Lateral heel callus
- Lateral ankle sprain
- Soft corn between the fourth and fifth toes
- Tailor's bunion (fifth metatarsophalangeal joint)
- Lesions beneath the first and fifth metatarsal heads (diffuse callus, not corns)
- Hard corn on the dorsum of the fifth toe
- Hip and low back pain

Quick treatment
- Protective padding to dorsal and interdigital lesions
- PMPs
- Taping for lateral ankle instability

Longer-term treatment
- Biomechanical assessment, gait analysis, sporting style and modification of training
- Footwear analysis, modification and advice; referral to a podiatrist

Compensated rearfoot varus

This is where the foot has obtained full ground contact by pronating at the subtalar and midtarsal joints for longer than normal.

Clues to look for:
- Mid-stance abductory twist of the foot
- Haglund's deformity (heel bumps)

- Bulging talar head
- Flattened medial longitudinal arch
- Lateral heel callus
- Lateral ankle sprain
- Hard/soft corns on the fourth or fifth toes
- Lesions or callus beneath all metatarsal heads
- Hammer toes
- Hard corn on the dorsum of the fifth toe
- Hip and low back pain

Quick treatment
- Protective padding to dorsal lesions
- Combined PMP with valgus filler pad
- Taping for lateral ankle instability

Longer-term treatment
- Biomechanical assessment, gait analysis, evaluation of function in sport, footwear advice, orthotic prescription
- Referral to a podiatrist

Rearfoot valgus (Fig. 3.21)

Definition

This is where the heel is everted relative to the bisection of the lower limb when the subtalar joint is in its neutral position, causing internal rotation of the leg and pronation of the foot.

Note: The forefoot is also angulated in this position but, unless the patient walks in sand, the ground reaction forces cause maximal dorsiflexion of the first ray in particular.

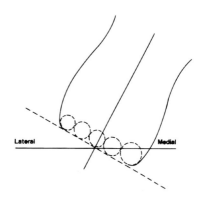

Figure 3.21

Clues to look for:

● Everted heel at mid-stance
● Low medial longitudinal arch
● Dorsal bump over the first metatarsopha-langeal/cuneiform/navicular articulation
● Lesion or hard corn beneath the first metatarsal head
● Medial pinch callus at the heel and first metatarsophalangeal joint area

Note: It is unlikely that this foot type will allow patients to compete comfortably in their chosen sport!

Quick treatment
● If the foot is mobile then use a combined PMP with a valgus filler pad and incorporate a wing shape around the plantar lesion
● Inversion taping
● Footwear advice and modification

Longer-term treatment
● Counselling on suitability to particular sporting activity
● Biomechanical assessment, gait analysis
● Orthotic prescription where appropriate
● Referral to a podiatrist

Forefoot varus (Fig. 3.22)

This is where the forefoot is inverted relative to the rearfoot, with the subtalar joint in its neutral position causing the foot to function in a pronated position from footflat onwards. It is possible for the foot to compensate by abnormally pronating the subtalar joint.

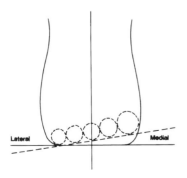

Figure 3.22

Clues to look for:
1. *Uncompensated forefoot varus*
● Propulsion off the lateral aspect of the foot
● Mid-stance abductory twist of the foot
● Mid-stance heel is *inverted*
● Lateral heel callus
● Spin callus beneath the fifth metatarsal head
2. *Partially compensated forefoot varus*
● May propulse off the lateral aspect of the foot
● Mid-stance heel is perpendicular or everted
● Mid-stance abductory twist of the foot
● Splayed forefoot
● Hypermobile first ray (moving when it should not during gait)
● Flattened medial longitudinal arch
● Usually, callus on medial heel border
● Lateral ankle sprain
● Tailor's bunion (fifth metatarsophalangeal joint)
● Diffuse callus over metatarsal heads plus hard corns beneath the fifth metatarsal head
● Hip and back pain
● Hallux abducto valgus subluxations
● Heel spur conditions
● Lateral knee strain
3. *Fully compensated forefoot varus*
As in (1) and (2) *plus*
● Bulging talar head
● Morton's syndrome
● Hammer toes
● Pinch callus at the first metatarsophalangeal joint

Quick treatment
● Medial forefoot wedge
● PMP
● Symptomatic padding

Longer-term treatment
● Biomechanical assessment
● Gait analysis
● Shoe advice
● Orthotic prescription
● Modification to sporting style and training programmes

Note: This is the most destructive foot type of all, because when the forefoot compensates by pronating to obtain ground contact, it has to bring the rearfoot also into a pronated position.

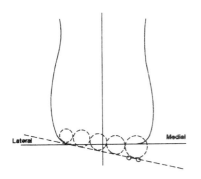

Figure 3.23

Forefoot valgus (Fig. 3.23)

Definition

This is where the forefoot is everted relative to the rearfoot, with the subtalar joint in its neutral position causing the medial side of the forefoot to come into contact with the ground very early in the gait cycle. The foot may compensate by dorsiflexing the first metatarsal to allow the lateral side of the forefoot into ground contact. If this movement is insufficient, the midtarsal and subtalar joints may supinate.

Clues to look for:
1. *Rigid forefoot valgus*
- Haglund's deformity (heel bumps)
- Mid-stance heel is perpendicular or *inverted*
- Spin callus beneath the fifth metatarsal head
- Lateral ankle sprain
- Soft corns between the second, third and fourth toes
- Tailor's bunion (fifth metatarsophalangeal joint)
- Tibial sesamoiditis
- Medial knee strain
- Hammer toes
2. *Flexible forefoot valgus*
- Mid-stance heel everted
- Splayed forefoot
- Hypermobile first ray
- Flattened medial-longitudinal arch
- Soft corn at the fourth and fifth toes
- Tailor's bunion (fifth metatarsophalangeal joint)
- Lesion beneath the second metatarsal head
- Hard corn on the dorsum of the fifth toe
- Hip and back pain

- Diffuse callus beneath the second, third and fourth metatarsal heads
- Hallux abducto valgus subluxations
- Medial knee strain
- Hammer toes

Quick treatment
- Lateral forefoot wedge to create full forefoot ground contact
- Allow a crescent shape around the first metatarsal head to accommodate any corn
- Stabilize heel with lateral heel wedge

Longer-term treatment
- Biomechanical assessment
- Gait analysis
- Orthotic prescription where appropriate
- Footwear advice and modification
- Referral to a podiatrist

Note: This foot type is a challenge to the therapist as it is quite difficult to achieve good results.

Equinus foot types

1. Talipes equinus
2. Metatarsus equinus

Definitions

Talipes equinus

This is a fixed position of the foot or part of the foot, showing a plantarflexed relationship with the leg.

Metatarsus equinus

This is a fixed plantarflexion of the forefoot to the rearfoot at the midtarsal joint complex (Chopart's or Shaeffers' joint; Fig. 3.24).

The foot may attempt to compensate for equinus by pronating the subtalar and midtarsal joints and/or lifting the heel at an early point in the gait cycle.

Clues to look for:
1. Partially compensated equinus
- Mid-stance abductory twist of the foot
- Mid-stance heel *everted*

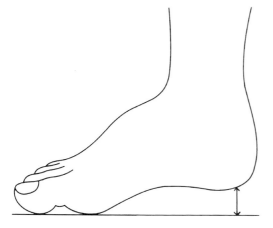

Figure 3.24

- Splayed forefoot
- Spin callus beneath the fifth metatarsal head
- Hard corn on the dorsum of the fifth toe
- Lesions beneath the first, second and/or fifth metatarsal heads
- Hip and low back pain
- Hallux abducto valgus subluxations
- Lateral knee strain
2. Compensated equinus
Same as above *plus*
- Bulging talar head
- Hypermobile first ray
- Flattened medial-longitudinal arch
- Midtarsal joint break (seen on X-ray as midfoot bulge)
- Early heel-off
- Hard corn on the dorsum of the fifth toe
- Lesion or hard corn beneath the second metatarsal head
- Lesions beneath metatarsal heads one to five
- Hip and low back pain
- Hallux abducto valgus subluxations
- Lateral knee strain
- Hammer toes

Quick treatment
- Heel raise in shoe
- PMP with crescent to the second metatarsal head
- Combined with a valgus filler pad if necessary
- Crescent pad to the fifth toe

Longer-term treatment
- Biomechanical assessment
- Gait analysis

- Footwear check
- Exercise programme for stretching, where appropriate
- Orthotic prescription as necessary

Leg length discrepancy

Definition

1. A small structural difference in leg length.
2. A functional leg length difference can be caused by the compensatory pronation for a varus or equinus foot type, or the persistent use of a banked indoor track.

Clues to look for:
- Difference in malleolar/knee or hip position when standing
- Excessive pronatory signs in the longer limb with supinatory signs in the shorter limb

Measurement

- Measure the leg length for both limbs with the patient lying supine. The shoulders, hips, knees and ankles should be parallel to each other
- Use the anterior superior iliac spine (ASIS) as a fixed bony point
- Measure the leg length from the ASIS to the midpoint of the medial malleolus
- Check each leg several times for accuracy
- If there is a discernible difference, then this will be a true leg length discrepancy

Quick treatment
- Insert a piece of felt into the footwear, 5 mm for up to 0.5 cm leg length difference, and 7 mm for up to 1 cm leg length difference. If there is a larger difference in leg length, then serial heel raising may need to be tried over a period of weeks, while the patient adjusts to the changed position

Longer-term treatment
- Footwear can be modified by incorporating a full-length lift to the outer sole, for a difference of up to 1 cm. This is the most effective treatment because the entire foot is short, not just the heel. Quality shoe repairers can

do this without the shoes looking obviously different. Both sports footwear and everyday shoes can be modified by similar methods. It is worth enquiring from the supplier whether the manufacturer will do this, or if the shop can provide this expert service.

Mechanics

● A change in the leg length will affect the musculoskeletal system and the patient should expect some discomfort while the body modifies position and function.

Summary

A range of structural and functional conditions of the lower limb are described. Clues are listed to facilitate the practitioner in their identification. Some quick and easy treatment programmes are presented, as are the longer-term aims of therapy. References are given at the end of this chapter, to help the practitioner in further understanding.

Further reading

Anthony R (1991) *The Manufacture and Use of the Functional Foot Orthosis.* Karger. Switzerland.

Neale D, Adams I (1989) *Common Foot Disorders* 3rd edn. Churchill Livingstone. Edinburgh.

Root M, Orien W, Weed J (1971) *Biomechanical Examination of the Foot*, Vol I. Clinical Biomechanics, Los Angeles, CA.

Root M, Orien W, Weed J (1977) *Normal and Abnormal Functions of the Foot*, Vol I. Clinical Biomechanics, Los Angeles, CA.

Spencer AM, Shadle JH, Watkins CA, Weiner S (1978) *Practical Podiatric Orthopaedic Procedures.* Ohio College of Podiatric Medicine, Cleveland, OH.

Chapter Four

The taping literature

S. Lennox

Introduction

Taping is not a substitute for treatment and rehabilitation but adds to and complements the total injury care programme. Each injury has unique features so techniques of taping cannot be completely standardized. It is important to keep abreast of new techniques and research.

Tape application

'Tape is the medicine, tension is the dose', a professor once cautioned as he demonstrated a classic low dye strapping.

Renstrom (1986) found that taping failure occurs at the skin–tape interface by shear failure rather than by breakage of the tape.

Mclean (1989) reported that the strongest adhesion is achieved by shaving the skin, applying tape adherent, e.g. tincture of benzoin, then applying non-stretch zinc oxide tape.

Hald and Fendel (1988) suggested shaving, not only for better adhesion but in reducing irritation and infection. They suggested skin preparations such as benzoin to protect the skin and provide increased adherent qualities to the tape.

Allergy to the adhesive materials may occur. Balduini et al. (1987) suggested 3 days as the maximum time for tape to be left on the skin, while Van Dam and Groth (1987) suggested only up to 24 hours.

Every piece of tape should have a purpose. The selection of tape depends on the skin, the sport, the athlete, strength of the tape, area to be taped, etc. Most authors agree that if the technique is not well-known by the trainer or physical therapist, it is best not to tape!

The mechanism of taping

Taping a joint increases mechanical joint stability directly but also may increase proprioceptive signals which are thought to be important in the regulation of the tone of muscles which normally helps to ensure stability. In a study by Konradsen and Ravn (1991), patients with a functionally unstable ankle had significantly increased postural sway and peroneal reaction time. This supports the theory that a proprioceptive reflex defect contributes to functional instability. Ten of the functionally unstable subjects were tested with and without ankle tape. The authors stated that: 'it could not be verified that a reflex enhancing effect of taping occurs through stimulation of cutaneous afferents'.

As effective mechanical support of an ankle by taping may only be for a limited period of time, does taping have a proprioceptive stimulating effect on peroneus brevis? Glick et al. (1976) claimed in a study that this may be so. If proprioceptive stimulation is the mechanism for successful ankle injury prevention in taping, would elastic tape be equally effective as rigid tape? Pirioli et al. (1988) used electrodynamographic measurements to study functional taping of the ankle, using non-stretch sticking plaster, non-stretch sticking bandages, plaster and Panelast or Porodress stretch bandages used alone or in combination. They showed that functionally sound taping was only created with non-stretch bandages used alone and mixed bandages employing graded elasticity. The latter was not acceptable to the athletes. Mclean (1989) stated that non-stretch tape has two advantages over stretch tape. 'The first is that there is one less variable in achieving the appropriate amount of joint limitation. Secondly, the elastic property of 60% extension tape is very short lived and contributes to the loosening effect of use'.

Compression

Compression is universally used as part of the immediate care of an athletic injury. Thorsson et al. (1987) showed that maximum compression (85 ± 8 mmHg) was necessary to cause immediate cessation of intramuscular blood flow in the compressed area. If maximum compression can be applied to an acute soft tissue it should effectively reduce or eliminate the formation of an intramuscular haematoma. Additional effects on the blood flow would not be expected by the use of ice.

Duffley and Knight (1989) studied the variability of using elastic wrap (with or without a horsehoe), an air-stirrup and the Edema II boot. There was a significant difference between the pressure exerted by the four devices and by the four trainers who applied the devices. Pressures exerted in this study were great enough to decrease or occlude venous blood flow, causing concern regarding adequate circulation. This shows that great care must be taken in applying compression.

Another study by Varpalotai and Knight (1991) gave similar cause for concern in compression application, this time by beginner and advanced student athletic trainers. Elastic wraps were applied to thighs and ankles and, although the mean pressures exerted were within recommended values, some individuals' pressures were frequently above this range. Pressures above this range have been found to compromise circulation or damage the compressed area. The ankles were wrapped using a combination of circular and figure-of-eight patterns, the thighs with a circular pattern.

Ruciniski et al. (1991) compared the effects of three treatment protocols on pitting oedema in patients with first- and second-degree sprained ankles. The three treatment protocols were elastic wrap, intermittent compression and elevation. Pre- and post-treatment volumetric measurements were taken of the ankles. The compression treatments produced increased oedema following treatment. It was concluded that elevation is the most appropriate of the three protocols in minimizing oedema in the postacute phase of rehabilitation.

Another study by Linde et al. (1986) investigated 82 consecutive athletes treated for ankle sprain with early mobilization treatment and (1) compression bandage and benzydamine 5% cream; (2) compression bandage and placebo cream; and (3) mobilization alone. A significant difference was found between those receiving benzydamine cream and compression and the untreated group (mobilization only). No significant difference was found between those with the compression bandage only and the untreated group. There was no significant difference in pain or function in any of the three groups. Capasso et al. (1989) investigated the compression action exerted on the ankle by adhesive and non-adhesive tapes. They concluded that only the adhesive tapes should be used for prolonged compression as these were still able to prevent swelling after 5 days.

Comparing tape to ankle stabilizers in preventing ankle sprains

A comparison between ankle taping and laced stabilizers (Miller and Hergenroeder, 1990) in the prophylaxis of ankle injury showed that taping with adhesive tape does offer protection against ankle sprains but that laced stabilizers offer an equal or greater amount of support. The laced stabilizers are cheaper, easier to apply and can be retightened frequently during activity. The authors stated that high-top shoes are better when the ankle is taped, although low-top shoes are better when a laced stabilizer is worn.

Similar results were reported by Rovere et al. (1988) in a study of 297 collegiate football players. They found that in a comparison of ankle taping with laced stabilizers the fewest ankle injuries occurred with low-top shoes and laced stabilizers.

The possibility that prophylactic ankle devices (taping, Swede-O-Ankle brace and Kallassy brace) may impair athletic performance was considered by Burks *et al.* (1991). They found that taping significantly decreased performance compared to ankles with no protection, but that there was less decrease with the braces (Swed-o-brace > Kallassy). However they did not advocate that the decreased performance from taping was a criterion for selecting a prophylactic support or brace instead of taping. Similarly, a study by Gehlsen *et al.* (1991) found that ankle joint prophylactive guards did limit force production, total work and range of movement, and that there was a difference between the three braces and the protective ankle tape support regarding the magnitude of ankle strength production and range of movement permitted.

Carmines *et al.* (1988) showed that in walking subjects (barefoot), taping served to reduce the range of ankle rotations in the sagittal plane by approximately 20% with a subsequent increase in the rotation about the metatarsal heads during the heel-up phase. Thus the taping served to shift the load-time history away from the heel and towards the ball of the foot. However, in a study by Kamill *et al.* (1987) it was claimed that, in normal running, the ankle appliances (boot-type ankle stabilizers and closed Gibney taping) do not appear to change or moderate foot function. In a comparison of inversion and eversion range restriction from athletic taping and semirigid orthosis before, during and after a 3-hour volleyball practice, Greene and Hillman (1990) demonstrated in 14 players that neither support affected jumping ability. They did find, though, that the maximum reduction in joint restriction due to taping, for both inversion and eversion, occurred at 20 minutes into the exercise, whereas only eversion was compromised with the orthosis at before and after exercise comparisons. They suggest 'that semi-rigid orthosis may be more effective than taping in providing initial ankle protection and in guarding against ligamentous re-injury'.

Gross *et al.* (1987) showed that ankle inversion movement after exercise was significantly greater than pre-exercise motion when taping is used and that semirigid orthosis limited ankle motion significantly more than taping, following exercise. The results suggest that the semirigid orthosis used in the study may be more effective in preventing ankle sprain injuries than athletic tape.

Foot taping

Two techniques have been identified that are effective in preventing excessive pronation with dancers (Lapenskie, 1985)–the Low Dye method and the longitudinal arch support.

A technique for a flattened transverse arch is described by Van Dam and Groth (1987). A foam wedge is placed beneath the second metatarsal bone, secured by a strip of tape. Further strips of tape are applied around the midfoot and then closed on the dorsal aspect.

A longitudinal arch support can be provided by tape (Van Dam and Groth, 1987). After applying an anchor strip across the transverse arch, a strip of tape is applied from the medial side of the calcaneum, around the calcaneum, underneath the sole of the foot, to finish at the first metatarsal head. Another strip is applied from the lateral side of the calcaneum, finishing at the fifth metatarsal head. Transverse strips close the sole aspect, and one transverse strip secures the dorsal aspect.

Macdonald (1987) described two removable supports–a medial arch support and a metatarsal head support. A dense foam or felt pad is sandwiched between two layers of stretch tape with the adhesive sides facing each other. The raw closure edges of the elastic tape are finished with rigid tape. Low Dye taping and longitudinal arch taping are both advocated for plantar fasciitis (Macdonald, 1987).

Ator *et al.* (1991) compared the support provided by Low Dye taping and Double X taping to the medial longitudinal arch, before and after exercise. Results showed that both techniques were initially effective in changing the height of floor to navicular height prior to exercise but both were unable to maintain this initial height after 10 minutes of jogging. However, they were able to maintain some degree of medial longitudinal arch support. This was not significant. It prevented joint motion at the end of range. For optimal support the tape should be applied as close to the start of the activity as possible.

Ankle taping

Most of the taping literature is on ankle taping. It is the most common joint to tape, yet despite its widespread use there are still questions on its efficacy and mechanism. Taping of the ankle joint is advocated at various stages of rehabilitation as well as in prevention. Many authors agree on the use of heel and lace pads, tape adherent and underwrap, but there are many techniques, including heel locks, figure-of-eight, basket weave, stirrups, etc. for providing support and injury prevention. These are adapted to the individual and the sport by the experienced taper. Several techniques can be combined to provide the eight-stirrup support (Moss, 1989), which is particularly used in injury prevention in lax joints and injury protection. The eight-stirrup technique replaces the Gibney strips and half of the stirrups. It can be modified for eversion sprains.

The treatment of ankle sprain in over 400 cadets at the US Military Academy is described by Ryan et al. (1989). They recommend open or closed Gibney strapping and, at a later stage of rehabilitation, a basket weave technique. The taping is completed by elastic adhesive tape, decreasing in pressure as it is applied distal to proximal.

Pope et al. (1987), using a model of a human ankle joint, tested four different types of ankle taping. Only the figure-of-eight with three or more wraps had adequate strength to withstand 8° of angular displacement (the level of pain initiation).

Balduini et al. (1987) advocated the open Gibney technique in acute ankle injuries for control of swelling and support. As soon as swelling decreases, a closed Gibney technique is recommended. Additional padding that may be incorporated into an ankle tape job, e.g. a J pad for subluxing peroneal tendons or a dorsal block in anterior impingement, has been described by Hald and Fendel (1988). Macdonald (1987) uses a compression support, the Spartan wrap, for acute ankle sprains. Under the underwrap are placed a horseshoe pad around the lateral malleolus and a boomerang-shaped pad, posterior and inferior to the medial malleolus. The centre of a 30 cm long strip of stretch tape is placed under the heel. Both ends are split to the tip of the malleoli and the two tails on each side are wrapped around the ankle. This applies tension over the two pads. A cohesive bandage finishes off the technique.

Ventura and Volpi (1991) described a rigid scaffold in the treatment of ankle sprain. The ankle is wrapped in an adhesive elastic bandage and then encased in a rigid scaffold. The authors claim it has significant advantages over traditional methods.

Van Unen (1987) recommends taping an ankle joint with elastic adhesive bandage (with hypoallergenic sticking material), and rigid tape applied to the other bandages. He claims that the principles of the bandage as a whole are neurophysiological. The tape is applied over the dermatomes.

Achilles tendon taping

Frignani et al. (1989) advocated taping the Achilles tendon with 'extendible' tape, but success will depend on its specific indication and the material and technique employed.

Van Dam and Groth (1987) described a taping technique using tape anchors on the transverse arch and around the lower leg at the tendomuscular junction of the calf musculature and Achilles tendon. Hypoallergenic stretch tape is applied from distal to proximal anchor over the heel. Another strip is fixed distally with tape. The proximal end is torn down the middle as far as the calcaneum and crossed over and fixed to the distal anchors.

Macdonald (1987) describes a similar technique but applies the proximal anchor of stretch tape of 7.5 cm width above the calf bulk and both anchors. She also recommends a felt pad under the heel and securing the technique with a cohesive bandage.

Medial tibial stress taping

Grant (1990) described a taping technique for supplying support to medial structures of the lower leg. The features include stirrups which are applied lateral to medial, heel locks which support the medial longitudinal arch and anchors to provide compression.

Macdonald (1987) suggested two techniques for supporting soft tissue structures after medial strain along the medial border of the tibia (associated with tibialis posterior strain and overpronation). Firstly, a strip of tape is applied from above the lateral malleolus, drawing it around the back of the leg, angling it upwards to finish on the anterolateral border of the tibia. This should be repeated three to four times. Secondly, a series of tape strips should be applied below the muscle bulk, providing compression, and in addition a pad should be placed under the medial arch and anchored with tape around the midfoot. These techniques should not be used for compartment syndromes or stress fractures of the tibia and fibula.

Knee–patellofemoral

McConnell (1986) described techniques to correct abnormal components of patellar position (e.g. excessive lateral tilt, decreased medial glide, abnormal rotation). Beckman *et al.* (1989) experienced limited success with patellar stabilizing braces and infrapatellar straps and did not consider them as a primary treatment. However, they recommend them for patients with a history of recurrent subluxation of the patella.

Sega *et al.* (1988) demonstrated significant reduction in pain in 20 patients with patellar instability using a dynamic adhesive elastic bandage. The effect was to medialize the patella.

Two taping techniques which relieve retropatellar pain (Macdonald, 1987) are the Crystal Palace wrap and the diamond wrap. Van Dam and Groth (1987) described the latter technique with additional vertical strips either side of the patella in rigid tape for conditions such as 'irritations of the patellar tendon or its sheath, as well as distortions of the patella'.

Knee–tibiofemoral

Van Dam and Groth (1987) advocated lateral and medial tape strips applied in a fan arrangement, anchored above and below the knee joint after varus or valgus strain, respectively. For medial joint strains, Macdonald (1987) described supporting strips of elastic tape applied from lateral calf to medial thigh passing under the patella, and from medial calf to lateral thigh passing above the patella, secured by mid-calf and mid-thigh anchors. The strips can be reinforced on the medial side with rigid tape. The tape may be pinched together for more tensile strength. A locking band should be applied around the patella, with a further band applying tension over the medial collateral ligament.

Ross (1987) modified the Duke–Simpson knee strapping to limit hyperextension of the knee in anterior cruciate ligament injury. A four-tailed piece of neoprene rubber is placed over underwrap from the popliteal fossa to above and below the patella, anteriorly. Elastic tape (7.5 cm) is used to make an anchor around the calf. This is continued upwards and over the lateral joint line; a circumferential anchor is made around the thigh. By continuing on the medial side, the tape is brought downwards and across the medial joint line, around the calf, then upwards across the medial joint line again. This is continued around the thigh and down across the lateral joint line. Pass around the calf again and pull laterally, then upwards and posteriorly. The author notes that closing the popliteal space is uncommon due to circulatory problems, but using the neoprene support appears to counteract the problem.

All the above knee tape techniques use underwrap and are finished using elastic wrap or cohesive bandage to cover the tape job.

Thigh contusions

Sim and Markey (1990) reported on bubble packing, a technique for protecting thigh contusions in the final stages of healing against further injury on return to sport. This involves applying tape adherent, a layer of underwrap 5 cm above and below the contusion site. The 5 cm bubble pack material is applied to the same area (use a 60 × 30 cm sheet of 5 cm bubble pack) secured by a 15 cm elastic wrap. The athlete can then wear a large pad over this to secure the bubble pack further. The authors advise that this padding can be used in other areas, such as rib, iliac crest and the brachii soft tissue.

Renstrom (1986) stated that tape only has the effect of compression on a muscle, therefore there is no stabilizing effect. Van Dam and Groth (1987) described a technique for lesions of the thigh musculature. Two wooden spatulas are placed lengthwise along the thigh and secured by eight to 10 circular tape strips ascending the thigh. The spatulas are then cut out and the gap closed by 10 transverse strips in tape.

Macdonald (1987) described two techniques for the thigh. Hamstring injuries require strips of 7.5 cm stretch tape. The centre of the first strip is placed on the back of the thigh above the popliteal fossa (protected by a pad). The ends are drawn forwards and upwards lifting the muscle. This is repeated, with each strip overlapping the previous one by half. The ends are secured with 3.75 cm non-stretch tape. For quadriceps strain, Macdonald (1987) advocated use of a felt ring over the injury with criss-crossing strips of stretch tape. These strips are anchored on a single vertical tape strip on the posterior aspect of the thigh. Alternate strips of rigid tape can be applied to reinforce the injury site.

Perreira (1987) advocated a foam doughnut-shaped pad, made with two layers of 2.5-cm soft foam and one layer of dense foam fitted inside a football thigh pad (by taping it directly to the skin), if a player is returned to action during the game. If the injury is severe enough to keep him out of the game, a further pad cut from 2.5-cm felt in the shape of a horseshoe should be applied inverted over the superior border of the patella and secured by a compression wrap. This will decrease gravitational swelling around the knee.

Wrist and hand taping

An injured finger should be splinted to the adjacent finger. Foam is placed between the fingers and tape is applied to allow interphalangeal movement. Hald and Fendel (1988) recommended that the index finger and the little finger should be avoided as a splint unless either finger is involved.

Collateral ligament sprains can be taped by applying 1.25 cm tape diagonally across the interphalangeal joint, wrapping the ends around the proximal and distal phalanx. Macdonald (1987) did not recommend application of tape to the nail as it may damage the nail bed on removal.

Hald and Fendel (1988) recommended that, for hyperextension injuries to the thumb, a check rein is applied between the thumb and the index finger, acknowledging that injuries can result to the metacarpophalangeal joint of the index finger. Macdonald (1987) suggested using a check rein too, but stabilizing the thumb to the rest of the palm of the hand.

A spica technique for self-application, using 2.5-cm tape, is suggested by Macdonald (1987) for hyperextension, and for hyperflexion by Hald and Fendel (1988). A more rigid thumb tape application for hyperextension is recommended by Macdonald (1987) using the palm and wrist as anchor points, supporting the carpometacarpal joints and the metacarpophalangeal joints with overlapping strips. Use of adhesive spray to the palm is essential for good tape adherence.

Hald and Fendel (1986) claim to limit carpal movement by applying strips of rigid tape around the wrist, extending 2–3 cm up the forearm. They add that a foam pad may be incorporated into the tape on the extensor aspect, in cases of dorsal impingement.

In hyperflexion and hyperextension injuries of the wrist, Macdonald (1987) advised a fan check rein applied to two anchors (palm and mid-forearm). Therefore, in hyperextension injuries the check rein is applied to the flexor aspect and vice versa. The amount of restriction will depend on the degree of protection required. This rigid tape technique should be wrapped in a waterproof cohesive bandage for water sports.

Elbow taping

Taping for this joint is most common with hyperextension injuries and medial collateral ligament sprains. A fan check rein is applied to two anchors of stretch tape (mid-forearm and mid-upper arm). Macdonald (1987) stated that the fan should be of rigid tape and that the patient should make a fist and contract the arm muscles when the anchors are applied. While the check rein is applied, the elbow should be flexed at 45–60°, to allow for skin movement on blocking full extension. Hald and Fendel (1988) modify the check rein principle for medial or lateral support.

Conclusion

There has been a considerable amount of research into taping in the last 5 years. The ankle joint taping techniques have been extensively reported upon. More research is needed on other joints. Although there have been studies into the mechanism of taping, some confusion still remains.

The application of tape is unique to each individual joint and injury type. Commercial braces provide general support. They do not fit as precisely as a moulded tape job!

References

Ator R, Gunn K, McPoil TG, Knecht HG (1991) The effect of adhesive strapping on medial longitudinal arch support before and after exercise. *Journal of Orthopaedic and Sports Physical Therapy*, **14**, 18–23.

Balduini FC, Vegso JJ, Torj JS, Torg T (1987) Management and rehabilitation of ligamentous injuries to the ankle. *Sports Medicine*, **4**, 364–380.

Beckman M, Craig R, Lehman RC (1989) Rehabilitation of patellofemoral dysfunction in the athlete. *Clinics in Sports Medicine*, **8**, 841–860.

Burks RT, Bean BG, Marcus R, Barker HB (1991) Analysis of athletic performance with prophylactic ankle devices. *American Journal of Sports Medicine*, **19**, 104–106.

Capasso G, Maffulli N, Testa V (1989) Ankle taping: support given by different materials. *British Journal of Sports Medicine*, **23**, 239–240.

Carmines DV, Nunley JA, EcElhaney JH (1988) Effects of ankle taping on the motion and loading pattern of the foot for walking subjects. *Journal of Orthopaedic Research*, **6**, 223–229.

Duffley HM, Knight KL (1989) Ankle compression variability using the elastic wrap, elastic wrap with a horseshoe, Edema II boot and air-stirrup brace. *Athletic Training*, **24**, 320–323.

Frignani R, Ferretti M, Romano D (1989) II bendaggio nelle tendinopatie dell'achilleo. (Results with taping in the management of Achilles tendon derangements.) *Italian Journal of Sports Traumatology*, **11**, 57–63.

Gehlsen GM, Pearson D, Bahamonde R (1991) Ankle joint strength, total work, and ROM: comparison between prophylactic devices. *Athletic Training*, **26**, 62–65.

Glick JM, Gordon RB, Nishimoto D (1976) The prevention and treatment of ankle injuries. *American Journal of Sports Medicine*, **4**, 13–141.

Grant JD (1990) Taping for medial tibial stress syndrome (shin splints). *Athletic Training*, **25**, 53–54.

Greene TA, Hillman SK (1990) Comparison of support provided by a semi-rigid orthosis and adhesive ankle taping before, during and after exercise. *American Journal of Sports Medicine*, **18**, 498–506.

Gross MT, Bradshaw MK, Ventry LC, Weller KH (1987) Comparison of support provided by ankle taping and semi-rigid orthosis. *Journal of Orthopaedic and Sports Physical Therapy (Baltimore, Md)*, 33–39.

Hald RD, Fendel D (1988) Taping and bracing. In: Mellion MB (ed) *Office Management of Sports Injuries and Athletic Problems* Henley and Belfus, Philadelphia, pp. 270–288.

Kamill J, Knutzen KM, Bates BT, Kirkpatrick G (1987) Evaluation of two ankle appliances using ground reaction force data. *Journal of the Canadian Athletic Therapists' Association (Oakville, Ont.)*, Spring, 3–7.

Konradsen L, Ravn JB (1991) Prolonged peroneal reaction time in ankle instability. *International Journal of Sports Medicine*, **12**, 290–292.

Lapenskie GP (1985) Foot taping for the dancer. In: Peterson DR *et al.* (eds) *Proceedings of a Conference: The Medical Aspects of Dance*. University of Western Ontario, London, Ontario, pp. 71–74.

Linde F, Hvass I, Juergenson U, Madsen F (1986) Early mobilizing treatment of ankle sprains. A clinical trial comparing three types of treatment. *Scandinavian Journal of Sports Sciences*, **8**, 71–74.

McConnell (1986) The management of CMP: a long term solution. *Australian Journal of Physiotherapy*, **23**, 220–221.

Macdonald R (1987) *Taping/Strapping: A Practical Guide*. BDF Medical Ltd. (i) pp. 20–21; (ii) pp. 34–35; (iii) pp. 36–37; (iv) pp. 38–39; (v) pp. 40–41; (vi) pp. 42–43; (vii) p. 13; (viii) pp. 12–13; (ix) pp. 14–15; (x) pp. 16–17; (xi) pp. 18–19.

Mclean DA (1989) Use of adhesive strapping in sport. *British Journal of Sports Medicine*, **23**, 147–149.

Miller EA, Hergenroeder AC (1990) Prophylactic ankle bracing. *Pediatric Clinics of North America*, **37**, 1175–1185.

Moss CL (1989) Ankle taping: the '8-stirrup' technique. *Athletic Training*, **24**, 339–341.

Perreira J (1987) Treating the quadriceps contusion. *Scholastic Coach*, **57**, 38; 40–41; 85.

Pirioli L, Mignani A, Mari G (1988) Valutazione tramite elettrodinamografia (E.D.G.) dei bendaggi funzionali delia tibio-tarsica nello sportivo. (Electrodynamographic (ED) evaluation of functional ankle taping in athletes.) *Italian Journal of Sports Traumatology (Milan)*, **10**, 235–242.

Pope MH, Renstrom P, Donnermeyer D, Morgenstern S (1987) A comparison of ankle taping methods. *Medicine and Science in Sports and Exercise*, **19**, 143–147.

Renstrom P (1986) Evaluation of ankle taping. In: Maehlum S, Nulsson S, Renstrom P (eds) *Proceedings from The Second Scandinavian Conference in Sports Medicine.* Soria Moria, Oslo, Norway, pp. 258–263.

Ross SE (1987) The supportive effect of modified Duke Simpson strapping. *Athletic Training*, **13**, 206.

Rovere GD, Clarke TJ, Yates CS, Burley K (1988) Retrospective comparison of taping and ankle stabilizers in preventing ankle injuries. *American Journal of Sports Medicine*, **16**, 228–233

Ruciniski TJ, Hooker DN, Prentice WE, Shields EW, Cote-Murray DJ (1991) The effects of intermittent compression on edema in postacute ankle sprains. *Journal of Orthopaedic and Sports Physical Therapy*, **14**, 65–69.

Ryan JB, Hopkinson WJ, Wheeler JH, Arciero RA, Swain JH (1989) Office management of the acute ankle sprain. *Clinics in Sports Medicine*, **8**, 477–495.

Sega L, Galante A, Fortina A, Viscontini GS, Bertolotti G, Benedetti MG (1988) L'impiego di un bendaggio dinamico nella instabilita rotulea in associazione al trattamento fisiochinesiterapico. (Association of a dynamic bandage with kinesitherapy in the treatment of patellar instability.) *Italian Journal of Sports Traumatology*, **10**, 89–94.

Sim D, Markey JM (1990) Bubble packing: an alternative technique for padding severe thigh contusions. *Athletic Training*, **25**, 163–165.

Thorsson O, Hemdal B, Westlin N (1987) The effect of external pressure on intra-muscular blood flow at rest and after running. *Medicine and Science in Sports and Exercise*, **19**, 469–473.

Van Dam B, Groth KH (1987) Taping for running: functional adhesive dressings for running events. *New Studies in Athletics*, **2**, 63–82.

Van Unen J (1987) La traumatologia in athletica leggera: il taping. *Italian Journal of Sports Traumatology*, **9**, 154–157.

Varpalotai M, Knight KL (1991) Pressures exerted by elastic wraps applied by beginning and advanced student athletic trainers to the ankle and the thigh with and without an ice pack. *Athletic Training*, **26**, 246–250.

Part Two

Chapter Five

Ankle

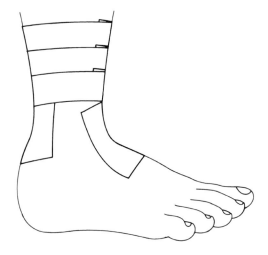

Figure 5.1

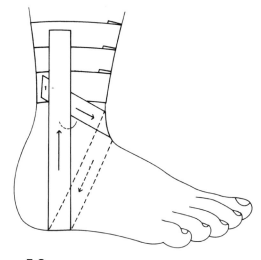

Figure 5.2

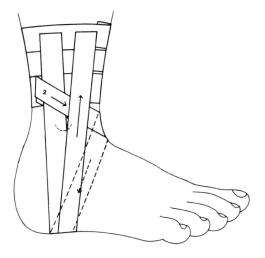

Figure 5.3

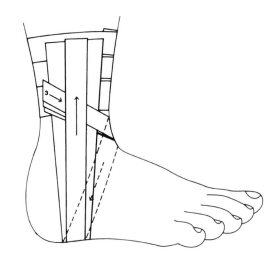

Figure 5.4

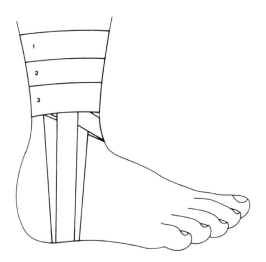

Figure 5.5

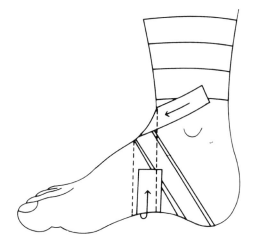

Figure 5.6

Preventive taping for injuries to the lateral aspect of the ankle joint

D. Reese

Indications	Prevention of injuries caused by foot inversion. Strain to the peroneus tendons. Slight or healing sprain to the anterior talofibular ligament and/or calcaneofibular ligament.
Function	To give support to the lateral aspect of the ankle by a combination of mechanical support supplied by the tape and its interface with the anchors and proprioceptive response triggered by the pull of the skin when supinating the foot during activity.
Materials	3.75/5 cm tape depending on the size of the ankle. Underwrap and/or two gauze squares with lubricant.
Position	Patient sitting with the foot over the end of the bench or the lower leg supported by a taping support under the lower leg.
Application	The patient should be clean, dry and shaved in the area to be taped. Start by having the patient actively holding the foot neutrally at the anatomical 0 position for the foot (or 90°). For patients who sweat profusely or who will be active in a wet environment it is recommended to use adhesive spray. Apply the underwrap in a figure-of-eight around the ankle joint, covering the lower aspect of the Achilles tendon and the dorsal aspect of the joint, or place two heel and lace pads or gauze squares with lubricant (one placed on the Achilles tendon, the other at the dorsal junction between the malleoli and the talus).
Anchors	Anchors 1, 2 and 3 should be placed starting approximately 5 cm distal to the belly of the gastrocnemius. Apply the tape so that it conforms to the natural angle of the lower leg. Overlap distally approximately one-quarter of the width of the first anchor. The bottom part of the last anchor should lie just proximal to the malleoli. Check to see that the anchors do not constrict the range of motion (Fig. 5.1).
Support	1. The first support should start just proximal to the lateral malleolus. It should be angled downwards towards the posterior aspect of the calcaneus and then pulled tautly upwards, covering the back half of the lateral malleolus and continuing upwards to the level of the first anchor (Fig. 5.2). 2. The second support starts proximal to the first support. The angle downwards should be directed so that, as it passes anteriorly to the medial malleolus, it should lie directly on top of the first support, continuing on the calcaneus to be pulled tautly upwards covering the anterior half of the malleolus, and creating a V formation together with the first support (Fig. 5.3). 3. The third support is placed in the centre of the first two. Pull tautly upwards covering the malleolus (Fig. 5.4).
Anchor lock	Apply three more anchors over the originals (Fig. 5.5).
Arch support	The arch support should start proximal to the *medial malleolus*. It passes downwards over the lateral aspect of the foot and then is pulled tautly upwards, finishing at the apex of the medial arch (Fig. 5.6).

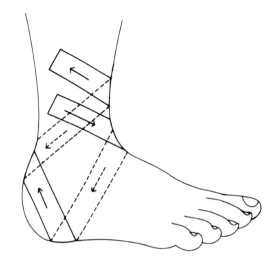

Figure 5.7

Heel lock	The lateral heel lock starts proximal to the *lateral malleolus*. It should be angled downwards towards the posterior aspect of calcaneum and then pulled tautly upwards, covering calcaneum laterally. It continues over the medial malleolus, angled upwards, and finishes parallel to the start (Fig. 5.7).
Check function	Once the supports have been applied, hold them manually in place and ask the patient if he or she is recieving the desired support. If not, adjust the supports before applying the anchor locks.
Contraindications	Application should be avoided when the patient has a swollen joint.
Tips	Best applied directly to the skin. When applying the supports be careful to keep proximal to the base of the fifth metatarsal.

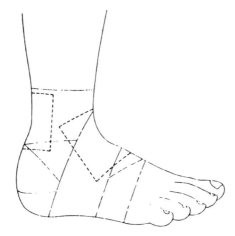

Figure 5.8

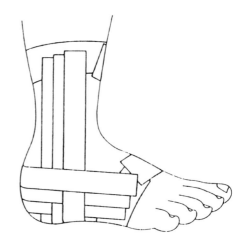

Figure 5.9

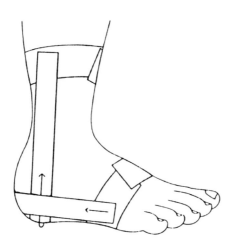

Figure 5.10

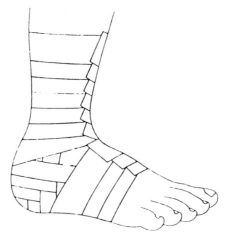

Figure 5.11

Figure 5.12

Closed basket weave for activity

R. Macdonald

Indication	Ankle inversion sprain.
Function	To support lateral ligaments without limiting motion unnecessarily.
Materials	Gauze squares or heel and lace pads, petroleum jelly, adhesive spray, underwrap, 3.75-cm tape.
Position	Patient sitting on couch/bench with foot and ankle over edge. Foot in dorsi-flexion and everted.
Application	Spray area. Apply lubricated gauze squares over pressure areas (extensor tendons and Achilles tendon). Apply a single layer of underwrap (Fig. 5.8).
Anchors	Apply anchors to the leg about 10 cm above the malleoli, conforming to the shape of the leg and to the midfoot. These anchors should overlap underwrap by 2 cm and adhere directly to the skin (Fig. 5.9).
Support	Apply first the vertical stirrup, starting on the medial side of the anchor. Continue down posterior to the medial malleolus, under the heel and up the lateral side (with tension). Attach to the anchor. (Do not mould to leg.)
Horizontal strips	Apply a horizontal (Gibney) strip. Start on the lateral side of the anchor, continue around the heel and attach to the medial side of the foot anchor (Fig. 5.10). Continue to apply vertical and horizontal strips alternately until ankle is covered. Ensure each strip overlaps the preceding one by one-third (Fig. 5.11).
Lock strips	Fill in with locking ½ fill strips between anchors (Fig. 5.12).
Check function	Is it supportive–not too tight?
Contraindications	Swelling–inflammation, bleeding.
Tip	Mould with hands to warm and set.

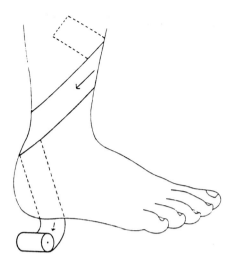

Figure 5.13

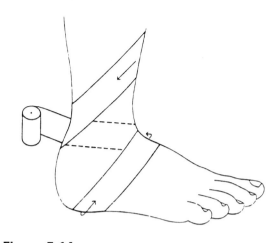

Figure 5.14

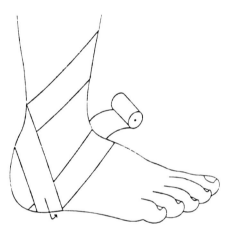

Figure 5.15

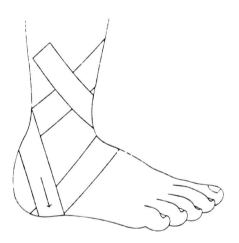

Figure 5.16

Reinforcement for closed basket weave
R. Macdonald

Indication   Ankle inversion sprain.

Function   To provide extra support with double heel lock.

Materials   3.75-cm tape.

Application
1. Start on the medial side of the leg. Angle tape down over the lateral side, behind and under the heel, pulling up and out (Fig. 5.13).
2. Continue over the dorsum of the foot, back over the medial malleolus behind the heel (Fig. 5.14).
3. Continue down under the heel, pulling up and out to the medial side (Fig. 5.15).
4. Proceed across the front of the foot and finish high on the lateral side (Fig. 5.16).

Tip   For the novice, two single heel locks are easier to apply–the first starting on the medial side, and the second on the lateral side.

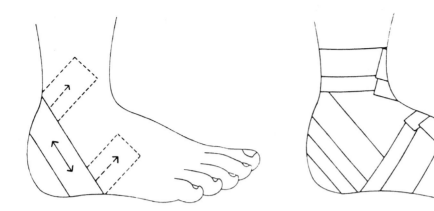

Figure 5.17

Alternative heel lock
R. Macdonald

Indication	Ankle inversion sprain
Function	To reinforce eversion taping.
Materials	3.75-cm tape.
Application	Apply three overlapping strips on the lateral aspect of the calcaneum, maintaining eversion. Secure with two anchors proximally and distally (Fig. 5.17).

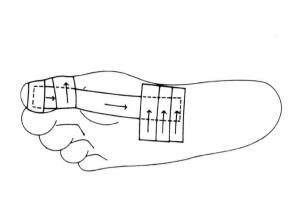

Figure 5.18

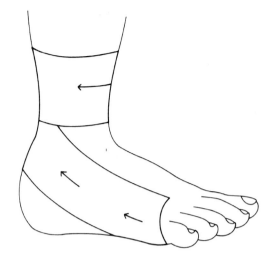

Figure 5.19

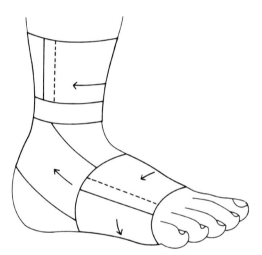

Figure 5.20

Ligament and tendon support
G. Lapenskie

Indication

To be used to eliminate the posteromedial joint line pain following inversion sprain of the ankle:
- Posterior tibiotalar ligament pain
- Flexor hallucis longus tendon irritation

Function

To reduce the tension on the posteromedial aspect of the ankle joint. To reduce the strain in the flexor hallucis longus tendon during gait.

Materials

Tape adherent, 2.0-cm tape, 7.5-cm stretch tape.

Position

Place the athlete in a long and sitting position with the foot suspended over the edge of the bed.

Application

1. Apply strips of tape from the plantar and distal aspect of the great toe to the mid-portion of the arch, ensuring that the plantar aspect of the metatarsophalangeal joint is completely covered. Anchor the tape by placing strips of tape around the distal and proximal phalanges of the toe, and across the arch of the foot. This prevents the toe from going into dorsiflexion (Fig. 5.18).
2. Place the foot in a neutral position and externally rotate the foot (on a transverse plane around an imaginary longitudinal axis passing down through the dome of the talus). Place a piece of 7.5-cm stretch tape on the lateral aspect of the foot; pull the tape posteriorly around the leg to anchor itself on the leg (Fig. 5.19).
3. Using the 7.5-cm stretch tape, anchor the tape around the foot and the lower leg (Fig. 5.20).

Check function

The patient should be able to run, toe off, without pain.

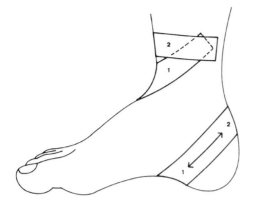

Figure 5.21

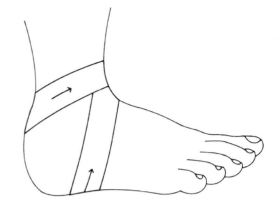

Figure 5.22

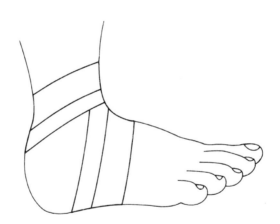

Figure 5.23

Calcaneal motion control

G. Lapenskie

Indication   Subtalar motion problems following inversion ankle sprain:
- Sinus tarsi pain
- Referred Achilles tendon pain
- Reflex peroneal weakness

Function   To maintain the subtalar joint in the neutral position by eliminating excessive calcaneal excursion.

Materials   Tape adherent, 2.5-cm stretch tape.

Position   The athlete is placed in a supine position.

Application
1. Position the calcaneus in the desired position.
2. To avoid excessive varus motion, cut a piece of stretch tape 30 cm in length, and place the mid-portion of the tape on the medial aspect of the calcaneus. Bring the end of the tape close to the metatarsal heads under the arch of the foot, up the lateral aspect of the foot, over the dorsum of the foot, ending the tape by wrapping it around the lower leg. The piece nearest the calcaneus comes behind the calcaneus, anteriorly over the lateral malleolus, ending the tape by wrapping it around the lower leg (Figs 5.21 and 5.22).
3. Repeat step 2 (Fig. 5.23).

Check function   Is calcaneum stabilized when the patient is running (rear view)?

Contraindications   None?

Tip   To avoid excessive valgus motion, start the tape on the lateral aspect of the calcaneus.

Chapter Six

Achilles tendon

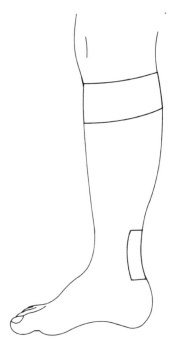

Figure 6.1

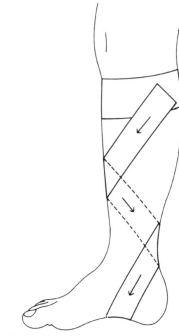

Figure 6.2

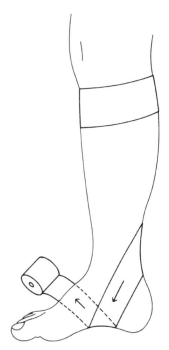

Figure 6.3

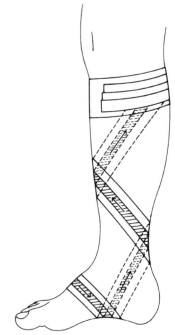

Figure 6.4

Achilles tendon taping procedure (Armstrong's Achilles spiral)

C. Armstrong

Indications

Achilles pain:
- Achilles tendinitis
- Mild Achilles strain
- Achilles bursitis

Function

1. To decrease some of the strain placed on the Achilles tendon during locomotion and leaping activities.
2. To limit dorsiflexion and thereby limit any stretching on the Achilles tendon.
3. To cradle and support the Achilles tendon.

Materials

Gauze squares, lubricant, adhesive spray. 5/7.5/10-cm stretch tape, 3.75-cm tape, 10-cm cohesive bandage.

Position

Patient in long sitting with ankle plantarflexed 20° in neutral; that is, neither inverted nor everted (Fig. 6.1).

Application

1. Shave the lower leg and foot.
2. Lubricate and apply gauze covering to the distal 10 cm of the Achilles tendon.
3. Apply adhesive spray to the skin area where tape will be applied.
4. Apply a 10-cm stretch tape anchor strip just below the knee and following the downward contour of the leg (Fig. 6.1).
5. Using 7.5-cm stretch tape, start at the proximal edge of the anchor on the anteromedial aspect of the shin, and angle distally and laterally across the shin, spiralling behind the leg to cross the Achilles tendon, passing down the inside of the heel (Fig. 6.2).
6. From here the tape goes under the foot and across to come up directly to cross the dorsum of the foot (Fig. 6.3).
7. Continuing with this roll of tape, head back under the foot to cross the last strip of tape in the middle of the plantar aspect of the foot. Angle back and up, travelling along the lateral aspect of the heel. Cross the Achilles and continue this spiral around to the front of the shin, angling upward and finishing on the proximal edge of the anchor on the anterolateral aspect of the leg (Fig. 6.4).
8. Run a second strip of stretch tape–this time 5 cm in width–centrally over and following precisely the path of the first strip.
9. Lock the anchor with three strips of 3.75-cm tape.
10. Wrap with a 10-cm cohesive bandage and leave on for 10 minutes to set the tape.

Check function

- Range of motion should be somewhat limited when the foot is passively dorsiflexed.
- The foot should tend to stay in neutral, that is, neither inverted nor everted.

Contraindications

Contraindicated if the patient has a predisposition to ankle sprain.

Tips

- Three symmetrical crosses should be formed in the midline by this taping procedure: (1) front of the shin; (2) over the Achilles; and (3) under the foot.
- Since this taping procedure makes the athlete more vulnerable to ankle sprain, one is advised to combine this tape job with an ankle support procedure when the patient is taking part in a sport that markedly increases the risk of ankle sprain.

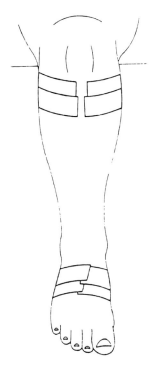

Figure 6.5

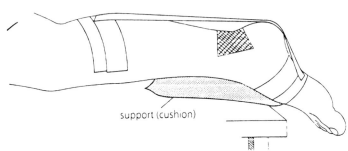

support (cushion)

Figure 6.6

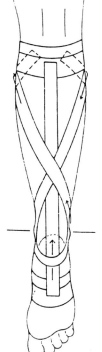

Figure 6.7

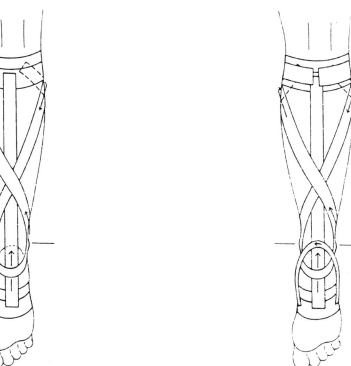

Figure 6.8

Achilles tendon support
R. Macdonald

Indication	Achilles tendon strain (peritendinitis)/calf strain.
Function	To restrict dorsiflexion of foot, thus avoiding overstretching tendon and calf muscles.
Materials	Adhesive spray, petroleum jelly, gauze square, underwrap, 7.5- and 5-cm stretch tape, 3.75-cm tape, felt, tubular or cohesive bandage.
Position	Sitting for anchors.
Application	Spray, apply protection pads and underwrap.
Anchors	Apply two 7.5-cm stretch anchors above calf bulk and two 3.75-cm tape anchors around midfoot (Fig. 6.5).
Second position	Prone with lower leg supported to flex knee and foot in slight plantarflexion.
Support strips	Apply a strip of 5-cm stretch tape from distal to proximal anchors. Exert slight stretch on tape. (Do not adhere to tendon; Fig. 6.6.)
	With 5-cm stretch tape apply to the lateral side of the proximal anchor. Mould tape to leg diagonally downwards to medial malleolus, passing under muscle bulk, under heel and diagonally upwards to attach to the medial side. Repeat if necessary (Fig. 6.7).
Lock strip	Secure each end to the top anchor with two strips of 3.75-cm tape. Apply a horizontal 3.75-cm tape strip from the lateral to the medial side of the foot anchor (Fig. 6.8).
	Reapply leg and foot anchors. Secure with a cohesive bandage and place felt pads under each heel.
Check function	Test to see if the procedure is functional for activity.
Contraindications	Acute condition.
Tip	For non-active procedure, place the leg anchors under the bulk of the calf.

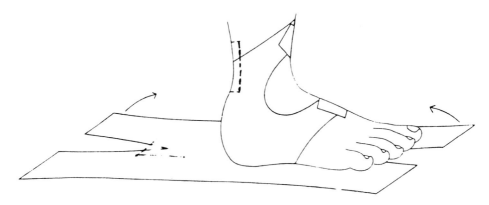

Figure 6.9

Achilles tendon support—simple self-application
R. Macdonald

Indication	Achilles tendon strain.
Materials	Adhesive spray, gauze square, felt pad 7.5-cm stretch tape, 3.75-cm tape.
Position	Sitting, knees bent with foot relaxed on couch.
Application	Spray and apply protection pad to Achilles tendon.
Support strip	Cut a 30-cm strip of 7.5-cm stretch tape and split the ends into four tails about 10 cm deep. Place the heel in the centre of the strip and wrap the front tails around midfoot. Wrap the other two tails around the lower leg above the Achilles tendon, pulling the foot into plantarflexion. Place the protective felt pad at the V junction of the rear tape split (Fig. 6.9).
Lock strips	Apply anchors to lock down the ends.
Check function	Ensure the Achilles tendon is protected.
Tip	Place heel pads under the heels.

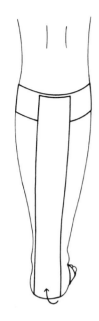

Figure 6.10

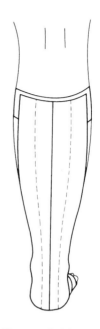

Figure 6.11

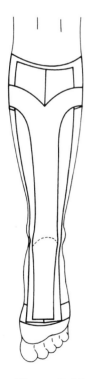

Figure 6.12

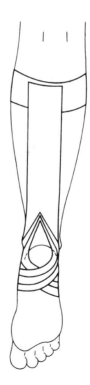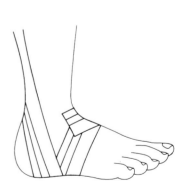

Figure 6.13

Achilles tendon support—three methods
O. Rouillon

Indications
1. Simple method–using stretch tape, non-weight-bearing, preventive.
2. To stabilize the rear foot, preventive.
3. Rigid tape method–for sport.
It is prophylactically better to use type 1 or 2.

Method 1–simple method

Materials
Gauze squares, lubricant, adhesive spray, pro-wrap, scissors–blunt-ended, 8- and 6-cm stretch tape.

Position
Sitting with leg over the end of the couch.

Application
Lubricated gauze square over the Achilles tendon. Adhesive spray on the leg. Pro-wrap from foot to top of calf.
1. Using 6-cm stretch, apply anchor around the foot, proximal to the metatarsal heads, another around the proximal end of the calf.

Position 2.
Prone lying
2. Using 6-cm stretch tape, attach it to the distal anchor on the plantar surface. Pass over the calcaneum and Achilles tendon and attach to the posterior aspect of proximal anchor, with tension (Fig. 6.10).
3. Attach two more strips to the plantar surface bisecting strip 1. Pass upwards to the proximal anchor with the inner edge travelling along the centre of strip 1, one each on the medial and lateral aspects (Fig. 6.11).
4. Using 8-cm stretch tape, attach it centrally on the distal anchor. Proceed as before up the posterior aspect of the calf. Before attaching, cut two tails at the proximal end, 20 cm long. Separate at the musculotendinous junction of the triceps surae; attach to the proximal anchor medial and lateral to the previous strips (Fig. 6.12).
Finish by repeating the original anchors (lock strips) proximal and distal.

Method 2–for rear foot stabilization

Materials
Two gauze squares for the Achilles tendon and the anterior foot tendons, spray, pro-wrap and lubricant.

Position
Proceed as for method 1.

Application
Using 6-cm stretch tape, apply two anchors.

Anchors
One around the midfoot, the second around the proximal calf.
1. Cut three strips of 6-cm tape, measuring from the proximal to the distal anchor. Attach to the proximal anchor. Cut two tails on the distal end 10 cm long. Split the tails to just above the Achilles tendon.
2. Apply the medial tail over the medial malleoli under the calcaneum, up the lateral side of the foot to finish on the dorsum. Repeat with the other tail, passing over the lateral aspect.
3. Apply the second and third strips in the same manner, superimposed on strip 1, moving anteriorly (Fig. 6.13).

Finish
Apply 6-cm cohesive wrap.

Tips
Three strips are cut before you start.

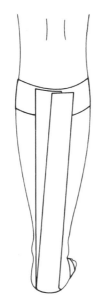

Figure 6.14

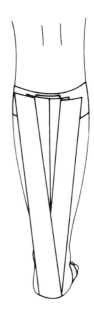

Figure 6.15

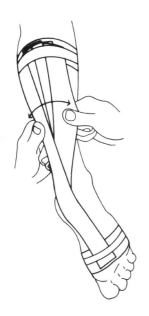

Figure 6.16

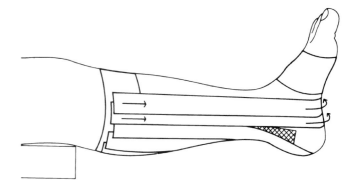

Figure 6.17

Method 3–rigid tape method

Indication

Active sport. The number of strips depends on the build of the athlete, weight, height and the sport and its constraints on the tendon.

Function

- Maximum protection of Achilles tendon.
- Suppress maximum stretch of Achilles tendon.

Materials

Gauze square, lube, pro-wrap, 6-cm stretch tape, 4-cm tape.

Position

Prone lying–leg over end of couch.

Application

Proceed as in previous methods–apply gauze, spray, pro-wrap, 6-cm stretch tape anchors distally and proximally.

Five to seven strips of 4-cm tape will be used.

1. With the foot in neutral, attach the first strip to the distal anchor plantar surface. Pass over the calcaneum and centrally over the Achilles tendon to proximal anchor (do not mould to the leg). *Note:* This first strip will be applied more laterally or medially on the proximal anchor to correct a rear foot, valgus or varus condition.
2. The second strip starts on the distal anchor superimposed on strip 1, passes to the posterior aspect of calcaneum, then diverges slightly laterally to attach to the proximal anchor covering the lateral half of the strip 1.
3. The third strip is applied symmetrically, covering the medial half of strip 1 (Fig 6.14).
4. The remaining strips are applied in the same fashion, fanning out on the proximal anchor by half the previous strip. Each strip passes over the posterior aspect of calcaneum and Achilles tendon insertion (Fig. 6.15).

Lock strips

5. Lock these strips in place proximally and distally with half-circles of tape.
6. Spread the strips apart, through their whole length–no wrinkles (Fig. 6.16).
7. Finish with a 6-cm cohesive wrap.
8. In certain cases, it may be useful for lateral stabilization of the ankle joint to apply two or three strips of tape from the medial to lateral aspect of the leg, attaching to the proximal anchor (Fig. 6.17).

Conclusion

Each one of the methods is for a unique situation. The three methods can be used for different stages of an injury. Choose the right moment to change techniques:

1. Non-weight-bearing.
2. Weight-bearing.
3. For sport.

The wrapping of injuries with an elastic structure (bati) stabilizes the rear foot and the part inferior to the Achilles tendon.

The frequently encountered sports injury, achilles tendinopathies, undeniably benefits from wrapping techniques during treatment and at the time of resumption of sporting activities.

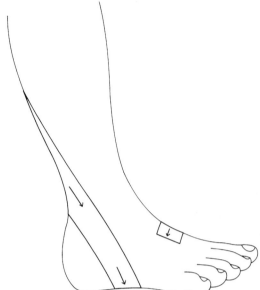

Figure 6.18

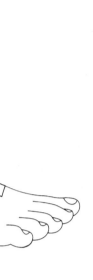

Figure 6.19

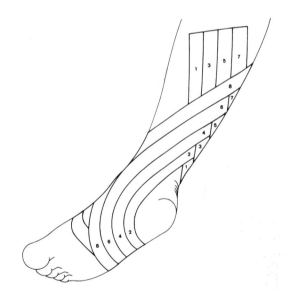

Figure 6.20

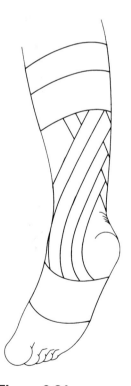

Figure 6.21

Ankle dorsiflexion and rear foot motion control

G. Lapenskie

Indication	Achilles tendon problems, subtalar motion problems: ● Achilles tendinitis ● Subtalar instabilities following inversion ankle sprains
Function	To control the amount of dorsiflexion of the ankle. To maintain the position of the rear foot during weight-bearing.
Materials	Adhesive spray, 3.75-cm tape, 7.5-cm stretch tape.
Position	Put the athlete prone lying with the foot extending beyond the bed. Place the rear foot in the desired position.
Application	1. Start a piece of 3.75-cm tape on the medial aspect of the leg at the distal third of the leg. Bring the tape laterally over the lateral aspect of the heel, under the arch, to the dorsum of the foot (Fig. 6.18). 2. Start a second piece of 3.75-cm taped on the lateral aspect of the leg at the distal third of the leg. Bring the tape medially over the medial aspect of the heel, under the arch, to the dorsum of the foot (Fig. 6.19). 3. Repeat the sequence three times in each direction, slightly overlapping towards the midline of the leg (Fig. 6.20).
Anchor strips	4. Anchor the proximal and distal ends of the tape with the 7.5-cm stretch tape (Fig. 6.21).
Check function	Is the tape irritating the Achilles tendon during gait?
Contraindications	Acute peritendinitis.
Tip	Heel cushion under heel.

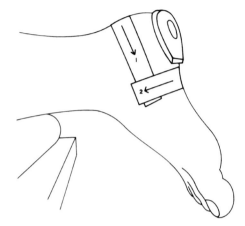

Figure 6.22

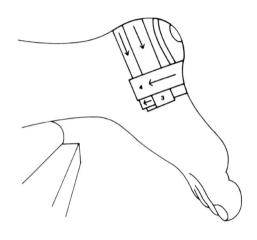

Figure 6.23

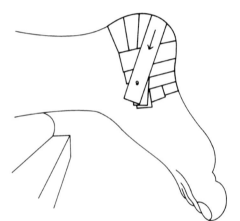

Figure 6.24

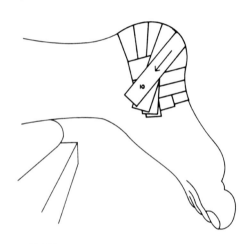

Figure 6.25

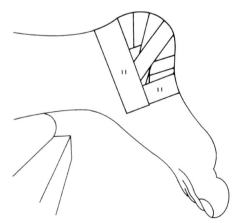

Figure 6.26

Heel bruise

D. Dixon

Indication	To alleviate pressure on a heel bruise–plantar surface or sides–caused by a kick or running and jumping.
Function	To compress the heel fat pad or to hold a sponge rubber heel pad in place.
Materials	Sponge rubber pad, adhesive spray, 2.5-cm tape.
Position	Patient lying prone with the foot over the end of the bed.
Application	Spray and stick heel pad to the base of the heel. Place a strip of tape around the calcaneum from lateral to medial, level with the insertion of the Achilles tendon. The second strips starts anterior to and below the lateral malleolus, passing under the heel and upwards on the medial aspect (Fig. 6.22). Continue twice more with this basket-weave–each strip overlapping the previous one–moving towards the rear of the heel (Fig. 6.23). The strips covering the posterior aspect of the calcaneum must be angled to conform with the shape of the heel (Figs 6.24–6.25).
Lock strips	Reapply the original anchors to finish (Fig. 6.26).
Check function	Can the patient plantar- and dorsiflex comfortably? Does the tape job take pressure off the bruise?
Contraindications	None.
Tip	A plastic heel cup may be used if available, to compress the heel fat pad. Apply three angled strips to the point of the heel conforming to the shape of the heel. Reapply the two anchors.

Chapter Seven

Foot

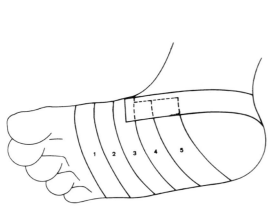

Figure 7.1

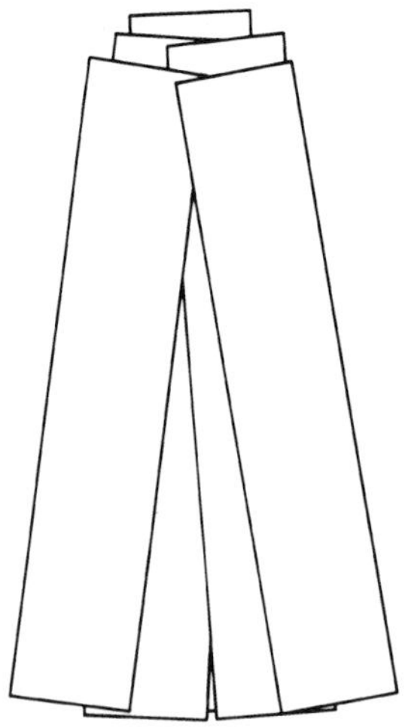

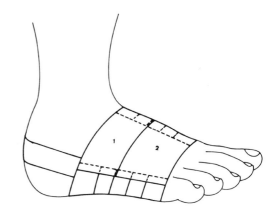

Figure 7.2

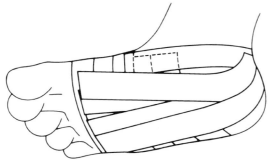

Figure 7.3

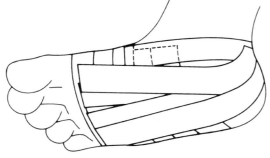

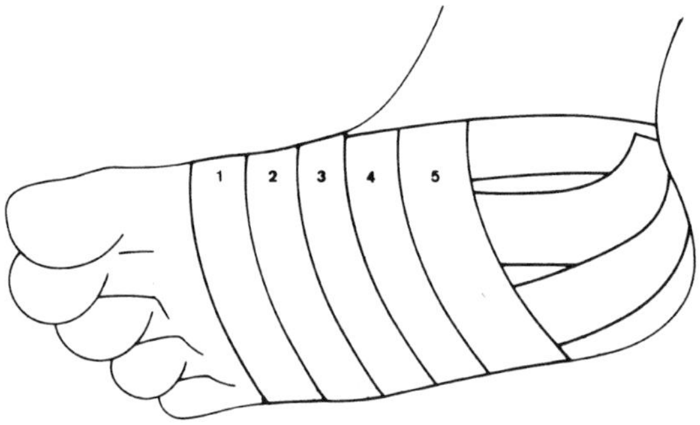

Figure 7.4

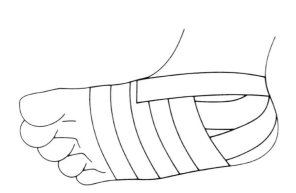

Figure 7.5

Figure 7.6

Longitudinal arch support
D. Reese

Indication	Sprain to the plantar aponeurosis or spring ligament, heel spur, strain to flexor hallucis brevis, flexor digitorum brevis, etc. These injuries can either be acute or chronic in all running sports and in jumping sports such as triple jump, high jump etc.
Function	To support the longitudinal arch mechanically and relieve the tension on the structural tissues to enhance healing. It can be used as a base for testing the function of support before producing foot orthotics.
Materials	3.75-cm tape, 7.5-cm stretch tape, adhesive spray.
Position	Patient sitting with the foot over the end of the bench or supported by a taping support under the lower leg.
Application	The patient should be clean, dry and shaved in the area to be taped. For patients who sweat profusely or who will be active in a wet environment, apply adhesive spray. The foot should be relaxed.
Anchors	Anchors 1–5 should be placed starting with the first anchor covering the forefoot at the level of the distal heads of the metatarsals. The anchors should be drawn up just to the dorsum of the foot and should not cross. Overlap proximally about half of the width of the first anchor. The bottom part of the anchor 5 should lie just distal to the tubercle of the calcaneus. The last anchor (6) should cover the posterior prominence of the calcaneus (make sure that the anchor does not go over the Achilles tendon). Check to see that the anchors do not constrict the range of motion (Fig. 7.1).
Support	Produce on a clean flat surface a fan of tape, the length measuring from the Achilles tendon insertion on the calcaneus to the toes. Start from a central point and fan out no wider than the forefoot, using at least five strips of tape. The width of the tape is dependent on the size of the foot (Fig. 7.2).
Support application	1. Start from the anchor (6) around the calcaneus and pull tautly forward to the forefoot. The patient should be relaxed: the therapist grasps the forefoot and pushes posteriorly to produce the desired apex of the longitudinal arch. Adjust the tension of the support accordingly (Fig. 7.3). 2. Cut away the excess part of the support, leaving ample attachment to the forefoot, where loading will be placed during activity.
Anchor lock	Repeat anchors 1–5, covering the first five. The anchors should start on the lateral aspect of the fifth metatarsal and be pulled tautly medially to enhance the tension in the arch support. Make sure to leave the dorsal side of the foot free from tape (Fig. 7.4). Repeat anchor 6 as before on the calcaneus (Fig. 7.5).
Finish	Have the patient stand on the taped foot and place two pieces of stretch tape over the dorsal aspect of the foot to hold the tape job together. Start proximally just below the talus. This will allow the patient to pull a sock on without the tape ends rolling (Fig. 7.6).
Check function	Check to see that the anchors do not constrict the range of motion.
Contraindications	Rule out the possibility of stress fractures before taping.
Tips	Instruct the patient that shoes should be worn to determine the effect of the tape job.

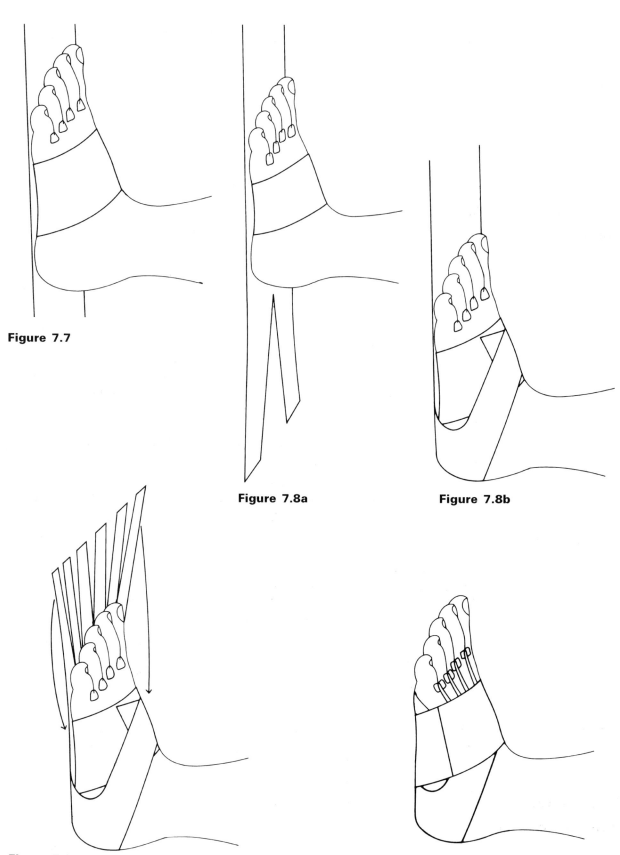

Figure 7.7

Figure 7.8a

Figure 7.8b

Figure 7.9

Figure 7.10

Longitudinal arch support (the Sanderson web)
C. Armstrong

Indications	Longitudinal arch pain: ● a fallen longitudinal arch ● wearing unsupportive footwear
Function	To support the longitudinal arch and thus take the stress off the joints of the midfoot and the soft tissue structures of the foot.
Materials	Adhesive spray, lubricant, 10-/7.5-cm stretch tape, 3.5-cm tape.
Position	Patient in long sitting with foot 20° plantarflexed, toes splayed.
Application	1. Shave the dorsum of the foot. 2. Lubricate between the toes and apply gauze. 3. Apply adhesive spray to the foot, including the heel; avoid the toes. 4. Apply a support/anchor strip (10-cm stretch tape) around the forefoot (Fig. 7.7). 5. Using a length of 10-cm stretch tape that stretches to twice the length of the foot, attach the tape to the heel so that the foot is in the middle of this length of tape (Fig. 7.8a). 6. Starting at the heel end of the tape, cut down the middle of the tape to just short of the heel. This will allow enough uncut tape to provide a pocket for the heel. Wrap the two split strips around the heel, crossing them over each other on the dorsum of the foot (Fig. 7.8b). 7. Then, going to the other end of the length of tape, make five equidistant longitudinal cuts down the tape (Fig. 7.9) so that, when stretched, the tape cuts correspond to the proximal ends of the spaces between the toes. 8. Bring the outside strips up from the plantar aspect of the foot. Make them taut and run them on both the lateral and the medial aspect of the foot. Then take the middle strips and stretch them and run them in the web spaces of the toes. These strips should end on the dorsum of the foot (Fig. 7.10). 9. Apply an anchor strip around the midfoot. 10. Wrap the foot with a 7.5-cm cohesive and leave it on for 10 minutes to set the tape.
Check function	Is the patient able to weight-bear without undue discomfort from the tape cutting into the web space between the toes?
Contraindications	● Severe athlete's foot. ● If long arch problem is second degree or worse.
Tips	● In cases where the arch needs more support than this taping procedure can supply, an arch support insert can be included. This arch support could be held in place with the midfoot anchors (Fig. 7.7). ● On a smaller foot, one might be well advised to use 7.5-cm rather than 10-cm stretch tape.

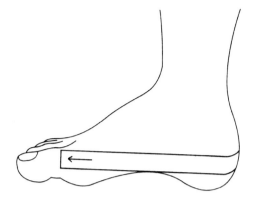

Figure 7.11a

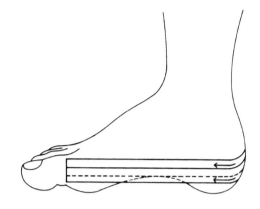

Figure 7.11b

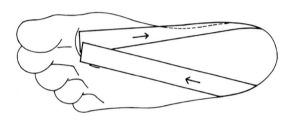

Figure 7.12a

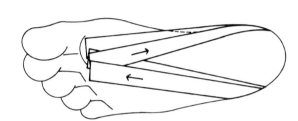

Figure 7.12b

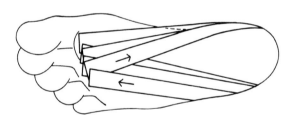

Figure 7.12c

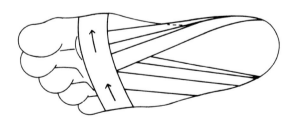

Figure 7.13

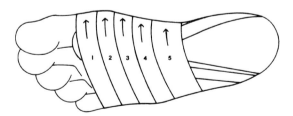

Figure 7.14

Foot support
G. Lapenskie

Indication
Foot pain, leg pain, retropatellar pain:
- Plantar fasciitis
- Tibialis posterior tenoperiostitis (shin splints)
- Patellar pain

Function
To support the soft tissue structures of the foot. To control the amount of longitudinal arch elongation (pronation) during weight-bearing.

Materials
Adhesive spray, 2.5-cm tape.

Position
Put the athlete in long sitting. Position the foot with the subtalar joint in a neutral position and the first ray in slight plantarflexion and have the athlete maintain the position (during steps 1 and 2).

Application
1. Apply tape adherent on the dorsal and plantar aspects of the foot and behind the calcaneus prior to positioning the athlete.
2. Start the strip of tape on the lateral aspect of the foot of the fifth metatarsal. Bring it posteriorly around the calcaneus to the lateral aspect of the first metatarsal (Fig. 7.11a).
3. Repeat step 1 overlapping the tape by 2.0 cm (Fig. 7.11b).
4. Start a strip of tape on the plantar aspect of the first metatarsal head. Bring the tape posteriorly around the heel, crossing the arch to return to the first metatarsal (Fig. 7.12a).
5. Start similar strips of tape under the second and third metatarsal heads (Figs. 7.12b and 7.12c).
6. Apply anchor strips. Start the tape on the lateral side of the foot; bring the tape across the plantar aspect of the foot. Push the thumb into the second, third and fourth metatarsal heads to splay the foot. While maintaining the play, bring the anchor strip over the dorsum of the foot (Fig. 7.13).

Repeat anchors, overlapping by one-half the tape width, to the tibialis anterior tendon (Fig. 7.14).

Check function
Is the patient pronating during gait? Is patellofemoral pain relieved?

Contraindications
Rigid foot? Pes planus?

Tip
Heel pad is sometimes beneficial (Cyriax).

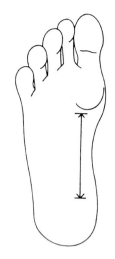

Figure 7.15

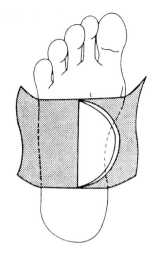

Figure 7.16

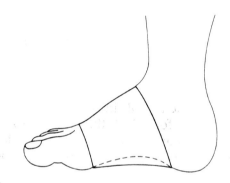

Figure 7.17

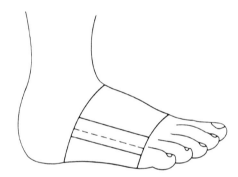

Figure 7.18

Medial arch support
R. Macdonald

Indication	Medial longitudinal arch pain or overpronation.
Function	To lift and support the medial arch and relieve stress on supporting ligaments.
Materials	Felt or dense foam for arch pad, 7.5- or 10-cm stretch tape, 2-/2.5-cm tape.
Position	Lying prone with the foot over the end of the couch.
Application	1. Measure distance from behind the first metatarsal head to the anterior aspect of the calcaneum (Fig. 7.15). Cut an arch pad to fit this size and of appropriate thickness to raise the arch. Bevel the side of the pad which lies along the midline of the plantar surface of the foot. Sit the patient up on the couch.
Anchor	2. Using 7.5/10-cm stretch tape, depending on size of foot, cut a strip to wrap around the midfoot. Apply with minimal tension, with adhesive side facing out. Ensure closing seam is to the lateral side of the foot (this avoids seams under laces). Place the pad in position with the straight edge along the midline of the foot (Fig. 7.16).
Support strip	3. Apply another strip of stretch tape over the first strip and pad–this time with the adhesive side innermost (Fig. 7.17).
Lock strip	4. Secure the seam with tape. Remove the entire support–turn inside out and close off the inside seam (Fig. 7.18).
Check function	Allow the patient to move support into position of maximum support.
Contraindication	Not to be worn in conjunction with a shoe containing built-up medial arch support.
Tip	Removable support may be placed in the most comfortable position by the patient. Talcum powder will eliminate tackiness on uncovered adhesive mass.

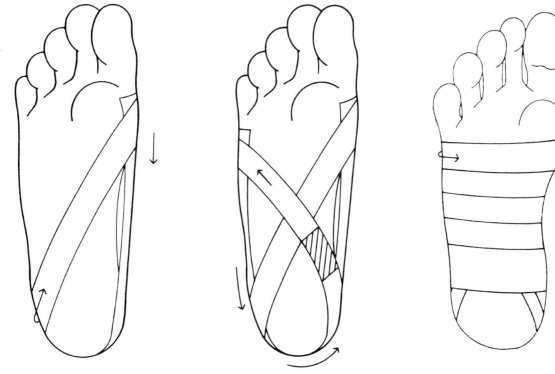

Figure 7.19   **Figure 7.20**   **Figure 7.21**

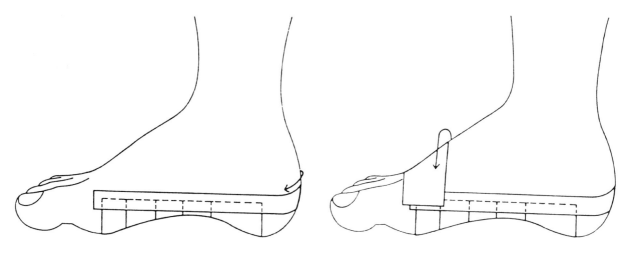

Figure 7.22   **Figure 7.23**

Plantar fasciitis support
R. Macdonald

Indication	Longitudinal arch strain–overpronation (plantar fasciitis).
Function	To support arch and relieve strain on plantar fascia.
Materials	5-cm stretch tape, 3.75-cm tape.
Position	Lying prone with foot in neutral position over the end of the couch.

Application

Support

1. Using 5-cm stretch tape start on the medial side of the foot, proximal to the head of the first metatarsal. Draw tape along the medial border, around the heel and across the sole of the foot. Finish at starting point (Fig. 7.19).
2. Repeat the procedure. Start proximal to the head of the fifth metatarsal. Draw the tape along the lateral border of the foot, around the heel and back to the starting point (applying tension as the tape passes over the plantar fascia attachment to the calcaneus; Fig. 7.20).

Cover strips

3. Fill in the sole of the foot with strips of stretch tape. Start at the metatarsal heads on the lateral side. Draw the tape towards the medial side. Lift the arch up before attaching medially (Fig. 7.21).

Lock strips

4. Secure edges by applying a strip of 3.75-cm tape from the fifth metatarsal head around the heel. Finish at the first metatarsal head (Fig. 7.22).
5. Stand the patient up. Apply one lock strip over the dorsum of the foot to secure the tape ends (Fig. 7.23).

Check function	Check that the great toe and little toe are not splayed. If so, release edges.
Contraindication	Rigid foot–pes planus.
Tip	Apply slight stretch to tape on application. A heel pad (Cyriax) is also beneficial.

For a sweaty foot apply the last lock strips around the whole foot, making sure that the forefoot is splayed (weight-bearing) before closing the ends on the dorsum of the foot.

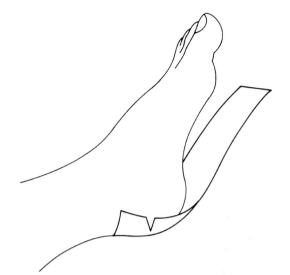

Figure 7.24

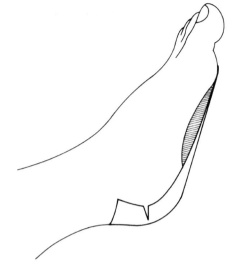

Figure 7.25

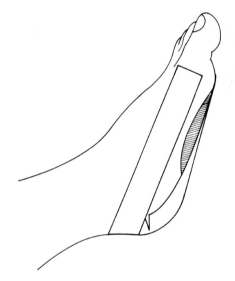

Figure 7.26

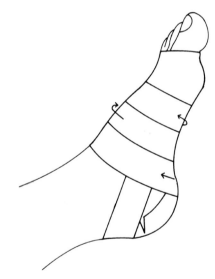

Figure 7.27

Plantar fasciitis taping
K. Wright

Indication Plantar fasciitis.

Function To aid in the reduction of stress on the plantar fascia and related foot strains.

Materials 7.5- or 10-cm adhesive felt (moleskin), 5- or 7.5-cm stretch tape, 2.5- or 3.75-cm adhesive tape.

Position Ankle placed in a slightly plantarflexed position.

Application

1. Cut the adhesive felt: measure its length from the metatarsal heads to the posterior aspect of the heel. With the ankle slightly plantarflexed, apply the adhesive felt strip at the posterior aspect of the heel and firmly pull towards the metatarsal heads. Once adequate tension is applied, press the adhesive felt against the plantar aspect of the metatarsal heads (Fig. 7.24). To eliminate binding, cut a V on both edges of the adhesive felt where the felt crosses the heel area (Fig. 7.25).

2. Apply a 2.5- or 3.75-cm adhesive anchor strip from the medial aspect of the first metatarsal, around the heel, to the lateral aspect of the fifth metatarsal head. Take care with the Achilles tendon (Fig. 7.26).

3. Apply 5- or 7.5-cm stretch tape around the midfoot area. It is preferred that this circular strip should begin on the dorsal aspect, go lateral, and continue across the plantar aspect to the medial portion of the foot, crossing the tape to finish on the lateral dorsum of the foot (Fig. 7.27).

Lock strip

4. Close off with a strip of tape.

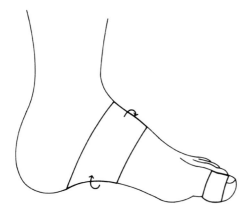

Figure 7.28

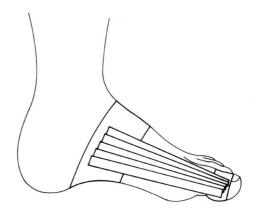

Figure 7.29

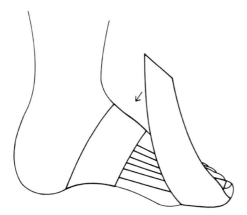

Figure 7.30

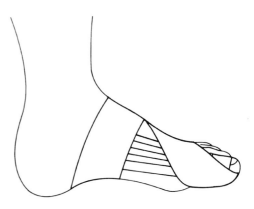

Figure 7.31

Great toe taping

Indication	Sprain to the first metatarsophalangeal joint (turf toe).
Function	To limit excessive motion of the first metatarsophalangeal joint.
Materials	2.5- or 3.75-cm adhesive tape, 5-cm stretch tape.
Position	Ankle should be placed in neutral position and the first metatarsophalangeal joint should be placed in neutral position.
Application	1. Cover the nail with a plaster. Depending on the cause of injury, the first metatarsophalangeal joint could be positioned in either a slightly flexed or neutral position.
	2. Apply two anchor strips to secure this procedure: (a) apply tape anchor strip around the distal aspect of the great toe; then (b) apply stretch anchor strip around the midfoot. It is preferred that this circular strip should begin on the dorsal aspect, go lateral, and continue across the plantar aspect to the medial portion of the midfoot, crossing the tape ends (Fig. 7.28).
	3. Use adhesive tape to form a fan shape (four to six strips should be applied to provide adequate support). Place fan-shaped tape from the anchor on the great toe, covering the affected area and ending on the stretch anchor at the midfoot (Fig. 7.29).
	4. Using a continuous strip of 5-cm stretch tape, apply a joint spica around the great toe and midfoot. This will aid in abduction of the first metatarsophalangeal joint. This technique should assist in preventing excessive movement (flexion or extension) of this metatarsophalangeal joint (Figs 7.30 and 7.31).
Lock strip	Finish off with a strip of tape.

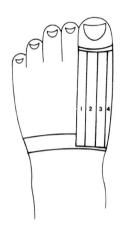

Figure 7.32

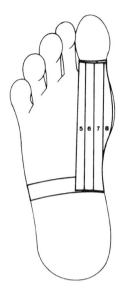

Figure 7.33

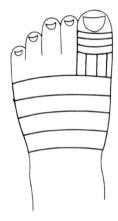

Figure 7.34

Turf toe strap
J. O'Neil

Function	To stabilize and support the big toe in sprain of the metatarsophalangeal joint.
Materials	Tape adherent, 2.5-cm porous athletic tape, 5-cm light elastic tape.
Position	The athlete should be sitting with the foot in a relaxed position over a table.
Application	1. Apply tape adherent.
	2. With the foot and big toe in a neutral position, apply anchor strips to the big toe and midfoot (Fig. 7.32).
	3. Apply four to six precut 2.5-cm strips (approx 15–20 cm long) starting at the big toe and pulling down towards the midfoot anchor, covering completely the metatarsophalangeal joint (dorsal and plantar; Fig. 7.33).
	4. Finish by covering the toe with two to three 2.5-cm strips. Cover the midfoot with 5-cm light elastic tape (Fig. 7.34).
Check function	It is important to check function. The purpose of the tape is to stabilize the joint; if this is not accomplished, pain will result–therefore the tape must be tightened.
Tips	1. If pain is only in one movement of the toes (whether in flexion or extension), prevent only that movement. This allows for greater mobility of toe.
	2. Do not put the toe at anatomical disadvantage – i.e. excessive flexion or extension–to prevent pain.

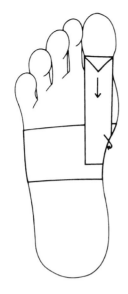

Figure 7.35

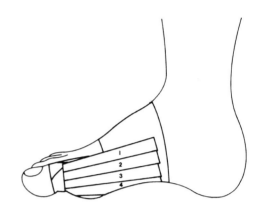

Figure 7.36

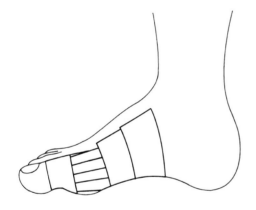

Figure 7.37

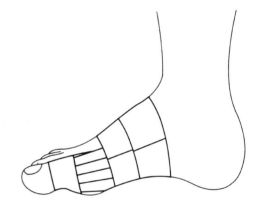

Figure 7.38

Turf toe variation
R. Macdonald

Indication	Pain in the plantar joint capsule of the great toe.
Function	To reduce forefoot motion and extension adduction of the great toe.
Materials	Padding, adhesive spray, 3.75-/2.5-cm adhesive tape, 5-cm stretch tape.
Position	Long sitting on couch with the leg supported.
Application	Place a sponge rubber pad around the proximal phalanx anchor with 2.5-cm tape. Place another anchor of 5-cm stretch tape around the midfoot. Cut a strip of 3.75-cm tape twice the distance between the two anchors. Fold the strip and cut a diamond in the centre just large enough to accommodate the head of the great toe. Reinforce this diamond by attaching another piece of tape–shorter than the first strip–sticky sides together. Grasp the ends of this doubled tape in both hands and pull over the toe, attaching the ends to the midfoot; anchor on both plantar and dorsal surfaces. There should be equal tension on both sides (Fig. 7.35).
Support	Apply three to four strips of 2.5-cm tape to the medial aspect of the metatarsophalangeal joint from the toe anchor, fanning out to the midfoot anchor (Fig. 7.36).
Lock strips	Apply 2.5-cm anchor to the toe. Apply two 3.75-cm anchors to the midfoot from the lateral dorsum, under the foot, to the medial dorsum–do not close (Fig. 7.37). Have the patient stand, then close the dorsum with two strips of 3.75-cm tape (Fig. 7.38).
Check function	Make sure the tape is not too tight in the toe web. Check that the toe is not abducted uncomfortably.
Contraindications	Swollen joint. If the patient cannot weight-bear.
Tip	Two to three strips of tape placed on top of each other before cutting the diamond make an effective splint for the joint. For a minor sprain this is all that is necessary, anchored to the foot and toe.

Chapter Eight

Knee

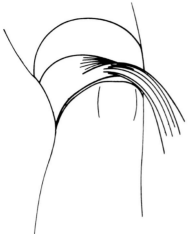

Figure 8.1

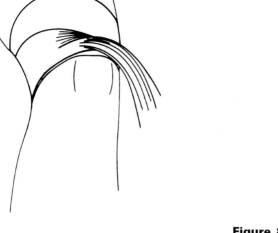

Figure 8.2

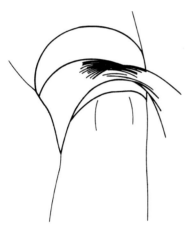

Figure 8.3a

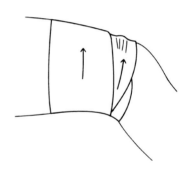

Figure 8.3b

Knee support
G. Lapenskie

Indication   Retropatellar pain:
- Patellofemoral dysfunction
- Jumper's knee

Function   Purported to affect the angle of pull of the quadriceps muscle. Purported to affect the patellofemoral contact surface. May change the stress distribution pattern through the patellar tendon.

Materials   10-cm cohesive bandage.

Position   Sit the athlete on the edge of the plinth with the distal part of the thigh extending beyond the plinth. Bring the knee to 40° from full extension and maintain the position passively by placing the athlete's foot on your thigh.

Application
1. Position the cohesive on the front of the thigh with one-quarter of the cohesive over the top of the patella. Anchor the cohesive in place by circumferentially wrapping the cohesive around the thigh until it overlaps.
2. When the cohesive passes over the superior position of the patella, put a twist in the cohesive by turning it 180°. Depress the superior pole of the patella with the thumb of the opposite hand and place the twist in the cohesive above the superior part of the patella to maintain the position of the patella (Fig. 8.1). Continue wrapping the cohesive around the thigh, placing a twist in the tensor over the top of the superolateral aspect of the patella (Fig. 8.2) and the superomedial aspect in subsequent passes (Fig. 8.3a).
3. Anchor the twist in place by wrapping the remaining length of the cohesive around the thigh (Fig. 8.3b).

Check function   The patient should be able to perform or run without pain.

Contraindications   Acute patellofemoral syndrome–retropatellar crepitus.

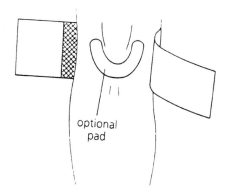

Figure 8.4

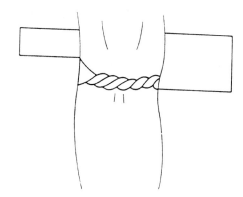

Figure 8.5

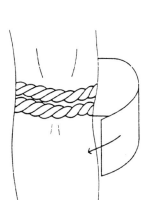

Figure 8.6

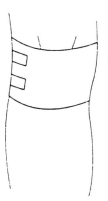

Figure 8.7

Knee support–Crystal Palace wrap
R. Macdonald

Indication	Retropatellar pain–jumper's knee–Osgood–Schlatter.
Function	To relieve pressure of the patella on the femur. To relieve stress on the tibial tubercle.
Materials	Gauze square, petroleum jelly, 5- or 7.5-cm stretch tape, 3.75-cm tape.
Position	Patient standing with the knee relaxed and slightly flexed.
Application	Cut a strip of stretch tape approximately 50 cm and place gauze in the centre.

Support strips
1. Lay tape on the back of the knee with the gauze square in the popliteal fossa. Mould the tape to femoral condyles (Fig. 8.4).
2. Split the lateral strip into two tails. Stretch and twist tails separately and attach to the medial condyle, passing over the patellar tendon in the soft spot between the inferior patella pole and tibial tubercle (Fig. 8.5). Repeat with the second tail (Fig. 8.6).
3. Stretch the medial strip across the twisted tails. Attach to the lateral condyle.

Lock strips
4. Close off with tape strips (Fig. 8.7).

Check function	Have the patient squat. Is it tight in the popliteal fossa?
Contraindications	Not suitable for those with rotated patellar dysfunction.
Tip	Best applied directly to the skin. Shave, wash and dry the skin. Apply skin prep or tough skin before taping.

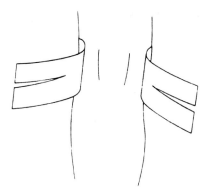

Figure 8.8

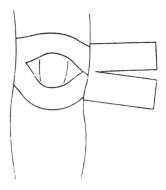

Figure 8.9

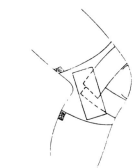

Figure 8.10

Knee support–alternative method–diamond wrap

R. Macdonald

Application

Using 10-cm stretch tape (Fig. 8.4) apply as above. Split both ends of the tape forming four tails (Fig. 8.8). Stretch the tails, apply firmly around the patella superiorly and inferiorly, interlocking the ends (Fig. 8.9). Close off with a strip of tape (Fig. 8.10).

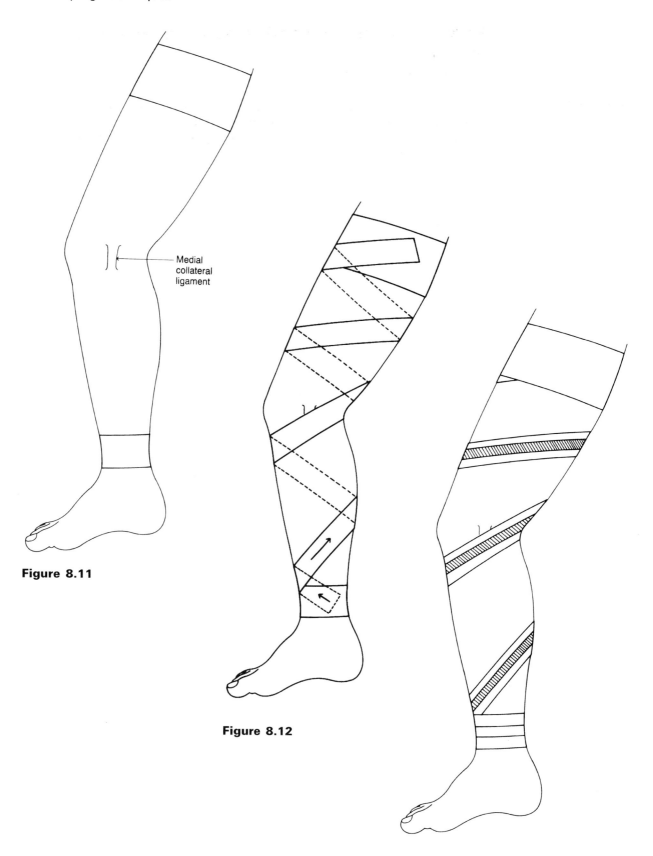

Medial
collateral
ligament

Figure 8.11

Figure 8.12

Figure 8.13

Protective taping of the medial collateral ligament of the knee (Kelly spiral)

C. Armstrong

Indication	Knee pain: • Mild sprain of the medial collateral ligament • Mild pinching of the medial meniscus
Function	To help align the lower leg on the thigh in a very moderate toe-in position and thus help take the stress/risk away from the medial collateral ligament and medial meniscus.
Materials	Adhesive spray, 7.5-/5-cm stretch tape, 3.75-cm white tape, 15-cm cohesive bandage.
Position	The patient should be standing with the injured leg forwards. The patient should flex the knee to the point where the knee blocks his or her view of the toes on the same leg. Then, keeping the foot flat on the table, force the knee laterally until the little toe can just be seen on the inside of the knee.

Application

1. Shave the leg from the groin to the ankle.
2. Apply adhesive spray to the leg, avoiding the back of the knee.
3. Using 7.5-cm stretch tape, apply an anchor around the ankle (Fig. 8.11).
4. Using 10-cm stretch tape, apply an anchor around the upper thigh (Fig. 8.11).
5. Beginning at the base of the distal anchor on the lateral side, using 7.5-cm stretch tape, commence the spiral coming anteriorly and medially (Fig. 8.12).
6. Angle around the calf, with the second circling coming up over the medial knee joint line and continuing behind the leg.
7. This strip continues to circle the thigh and ends on the proximal edge of the proximal anchor on the medial side (Fig. 8.12).
8. Copy this spiral with a strip of 5-cm stretch tape.
9. Cover the distal anchor with three strips of 3.75-cm tape.
10. Cover the proximal anchor with another strip of 10-cm stretch tape (Fig. 8.13).
11. Wrap a 15-cm cohesive bandage over this tape job and leave it on for 10 minutes to set the tape.

Check function	When the patient runs, the lower leg should tend to toe-in.
Contraindications	• If the medial collateral ligament sprain gives pain on weight-bearing. • If there is any discomfort during controlled running activities. • If the knee is considered unstable.
Tips	The stretch tape should be at 90% of full tension for the spiral.

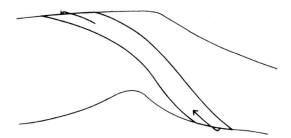

Figure 8.14

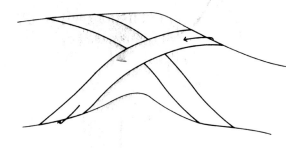

Figure 8.15

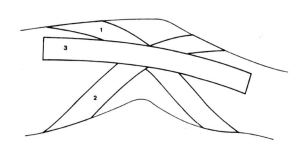

Figure 8.16

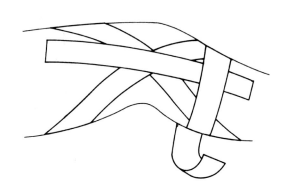

Figure 8.17

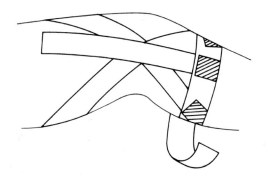

Figure 8.18

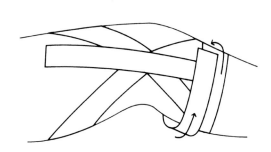

Figure 8.19

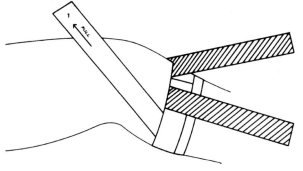

Figure 8.20

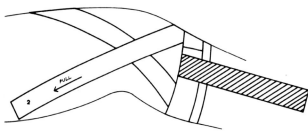

Figure 8.21

Proprioceptive taping for the medial collateral ligament of the knee
D. Reese

Indication	Sprain to the medial collateral ligament where passive stability is intact. Quadriceps inhibition by a pain reflex at specific points in the range of motion can cause further insult to the knee joint.
Function	To produce a slight mechanical support for injuries caused by forces applied to the lateral side of the knee resulting in injury to the medial side of the knee. To increase awareness of muscle activity around the knee throughout a normal range of motion directed by traction on the skin.
Materials	7.5-cm stretch tape, adhesive spray.
Position	Patient standing with relaxed and slightly flexed knee with a roll of tape under the heel.
Application	The leg should be clean, dry and shaved in the area to be taped. For patients who sweat profusely or who wil be active in a wet environment adhesive spray is recommended.

Support

1. Cut three 45-cm strips of stretch tape and hang them on the taping table.
2. Apply the first strip without tension, starting about 15–20 cm below the knee joint line lateral of the posterior midline. Direct the strip over the centre of the medial joint line and upwards above the patella over the anterior midline approximately 15–20 cm above the joint line (Fig. 8.14).
3. Apply the second strip without tension starting about 15–20 cm below the joint line lateral to the anterior midline. Direct the strip upwards below the patella and over the middle of the medial joint line crossing the first strip, continue upwards towards the posterior midline on the thigh approximately 15–20 cm above the joint line (Fig. 8.15).
4. Apply the third strip without tension through the middle of the X formed by the first two strips (Fig. 8.16).

Lower locking anchor

1. Place an anchor around the lower leg, leaving about 2.5 cm of the three supports sticking out underneath. Do not cut the anchor yet (Fig. 8.17).
2. Fold the three supports up on to the anchor and continue the anchor around the leg to cover the overlap (Fig. 8.18). *Continue to spiral upwards* to the tibial tubercle and cut the anchor. Make sure that no tape is in the popliteal fossa (Fig. 8.19).

Support

1. Fold down all three supports.
2. Rotate the foot and hip outwards. Take a firm grip on the lower anchor and pull out 90% of the elasticity in the first support, following the originally applied direction. Have the patient hold the end tension (Fig. 8.20).
3. Rotate the foot and hip inwards. Take a firm grip on the lower anchor and pull out 90% of the elasticity in the second support, following the originally applied direction. Have the patient hold the end tension (Fig. 8.21).

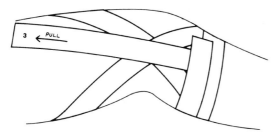

Figure 8.22

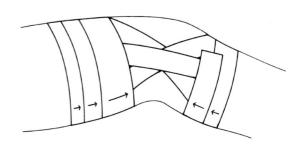

Figure 8.23

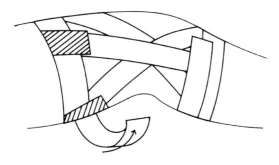

Figure 8.24

Figure 8.25

4. Return to the neutral position for the foot and hip. Take a firm grip on the lower anchor and pull out 90% of the elasticity in the third support through the middle of the X formed by the first two pieces (Fig. 8.22).

Upper locking anchor

1. The upper edge of the anchor that encircles the thigh should be about 15 cm above the medial joint line. This should leave about 12–15 cm of the three tensioned supports sticking out above the anchor. Do not cut the anchor yet (Fig. 8.23).
2. Fold the three supports downwards, retaining the tension on to the anchor, and continue the anchor around the thigh to cover the overlap (Fig. 8.24). *Continue to spiral downwards* to the top of the patella and cut the anchor. Make sure that tape is not in the popliteal fossa (Fig. 8.25).

Check function Functional stability–proprioceptive awareness.

Contraindication Rule out the possibility of passive instability, muscle atrophy and locking of the joint.

Tip Make sure that the knee is slightly bent when applying the taping. Make sure that no tape is in the popliteal space or over the patella. Application is best applied directly to the skin.

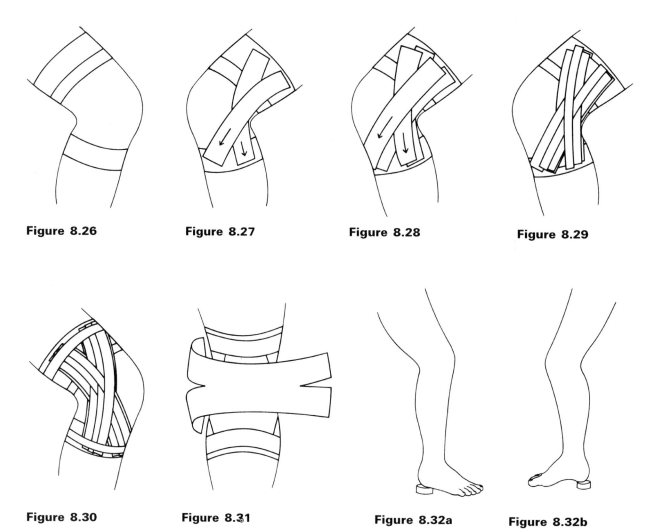

Figure 8.26 **Figure 8.27** **Figure 8.28** **Figure 8.29**

Figure 8.30 **Figure 8.31** **Figure 8.32a** **Figure 8.32b**

Sprain of the lateral collateral ligament
O. Rouillon

Function   To provide basic lateral stabilization of the knee.

Materials   Lubricant, gauze squares, adhesive spray, two rolls of 6-cm stretch tape, 15-cm stretch tape, 3.75-cm tape.

Position   The patient is standing with the knee in 15° flexion and the roll of tape under the heel. The leg is pushed laterally. Apply the gauze with lubricant to the popliteal fossa, apply adhesive spray and pro-wrap.

Application

1. Using 6-cm stretch tape apply two anchors to the lower third of the thigh and one anchor at the tibial tubercle (Fig. 8.26).
2. Using 6-cm stretch tape, apply a diagonal strip from the anteromedial aspect of the proximal anchor to the posteriormedial aspect of the distal anchor.
3. The second symmetrical strip crosses the first at the centre of the medial joint line (Fig. 8.27).
4. Repeat this sequence with two more strips overlapping the previous strips by one-half anteriorly (Fig. 8.28).
5. Repeat the same sequence on the lateral knee joint.
6. Using six strips of 3.75-cm tape, apply a symmetrical montage–on top of the previous strips–with tension on the medial and lateral aspects of the knee joint (Fig. 8.29).
7. Lock the tape job in place with incomplete circles of tape (Fig. 8.30).

To protect the popliteal fossa, using a strip of 15-cm stretch tape, cut four tails on either end. Place the lubricated gauze square in the centre. Close the tails above and below the patella (Fig. 8.31).

Finish with 6-cm stretch tape by reapplying the original anchors.

Figure 8.32(a) shows the position of the leg for figures 8.26 and 8.30, and Figure 8.32(b) shows the position of the leg for figure 8.27.

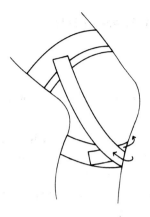

Figure 8.33

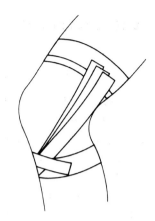

Figure 8.34

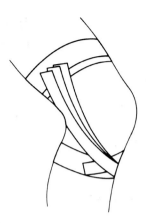

Figure 8.35

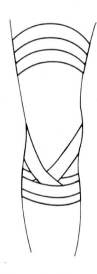

Figure 8.36a

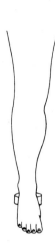

Figure 8.36b

Knee variation to reinforce the previous basic tape job

O. Rouillon

Function	To stabilize anterior drawer; to limit medial/lateral rotation of femur or tibia; to limit hyperextension.
Materials	Prowrap, 8-cm stretch tape, 3.75-cm tape.
Position	The knee is flexed with the heel on the tape roll and the leg in neutral position.
Application	Using 8-cm stretch tape, apply two anchors to the lower third of the thigh and one anchor distal to the tibial tubercle. Use one strip of 3.75-cm tape 25–30 cm long. Starting on the anterolateral aspect of the distal anchor, pass with full tension anteriorly below the tibial tubercle and diagonally upwards to the proximal anchor. Apply the second strip on the lateral aspect with the same tension (Fig. 8.33).

Apply two more strips medially and laterally over the initial strips superimposed on the inferior tails, fanning out and overlapping by one-half, to attach to the proximal anchor (Figs 8.34 and 8.35). Lock these six strips in place with tape above and below without tension (Fig. 8.36a).

Figure 8.36b shows the position of the leg for the taping procedure.

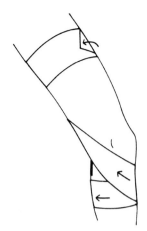

Figure 8.37

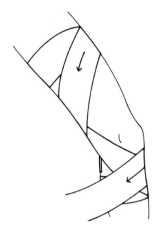

Figure 8.38

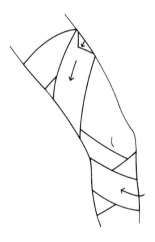

Figure 8.39

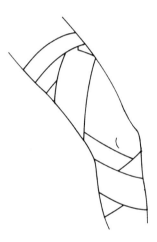

Figure 8.40

Anterior cruciate taping
K. Wright

Indication	Sprain to the anterior cruciate ligament of the knee.
Function	To provide support and stability to the anterior cruciate ligament of the knee.
Materials	5-cm adhesive tape, 7.5-cm stretch tape, gauze square with lubricant.
Position	Knee and hip joints should be positioned in slight flexion.

Application

1. Gauze with lubricant should be applied to the posterior aspect (popliteal space) of the knee joint. Apply an anchor strip of 7.5-cm stretch tape around the upper third of the thigh. Caution should be exercised in the application of tape so that the popliteal space is not compressed.
2. Using the 7.5-cm stretch tape begin on the lateral aspect of the lower leg, approximately 2.5 cm below the patella. Encircle the lower leg: move anteriorly, then to the medial side, continue to the posterior aspect and return to the lateral side. Angle the tape below the patella, cross the medial joint line and popliteal space, and spiral up to the anterior portion of the anchor on the upper thigh (Fig. 8.37).
3. The next strip of tape will begin on the anterior aspect of the proximal anchor, crossing the medial portion of the thigh, covering the popliteal space. Encircle the lower leg, cross the popliteal space again, and finish by spiralling up to the anterior aspect of the proximal anchor on the thigh (Fig. 8.38).
4. Repeat step 3 (Fig. 8.39).
5. Secure this technique by applying an anchor of 5-cm adhesive tape over the anchor on the thigh (Fig. 8.40).

Chapter Nine

Shoulder girdle

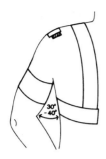

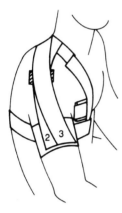

Figure 9.1

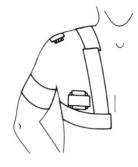

Figure 9.2

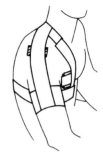

Figure 9.3

Figure 9.4

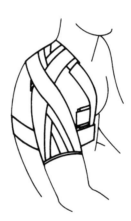

Figure 9.5

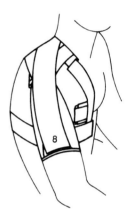

Figure 9.6

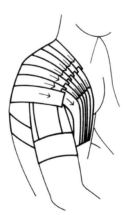

Figure 9.7

Subluxation of the acromioclavicular joint
O. Rouillon

Indications   Stretched acromioclavicular ligament–subluxations grades 1 and 2 only.

Function   To support stretched ligaments–protect and support acromioclavicular joint disruption grades 1 and 2.

Materials   Spray, gauze square, lubricant, felt pad 10 × 10 cm, pro-wrap, 8-cm stretch tape/10-cm cohesive bandage, 3.75-cm tape.

Position   The patient is sitting with the arm abducted 30–45° and resting on the table.

Application   Place the lubricant and protection pad over the nipple, anchored with 3.75-cm tape. Spray the area to be taped. Apply 8-cm stretch tape anchor around the upper arm.

Thoracic anchors   Apply two half-anchors on the shoulders with 3.75-cm tape.
1. Apply the tape paravertebral to the posterior aspect of the clavicle (Fig. 9.1).
2. Apply tape parallel to the sternum on the anterior aspect, overlapping the first by 5–7 cm.
3. Apply anchors around the thorax two half-circles posteriorly and anteriorly without tension (Fig. 9.2).

Support strips   Place a protection pad on the acromioclavicular joint for comfort–six to eight strips of 3.75-cm tape, applied from the arm anchor to the thoracic anchor under light tension, following this sequence:
1. The first strip is applied along the longitudinal axis of the arm over the acromioclavicular joint (Fig. 9.3).
2. The second strip starts on the posterior half of strip 1 and passes over the shoulder and diagonally forwards to the shoulder anchor (Fig. 9.4).
3. The third strip starts on the anterior half of strip 1 on the arm anchor and passes diagonally posterior to attach to the shoulder anchor (Fig. 9.4). Apply four more strips in this fashion, fanning out by half the tape width on both anchors (Fig. 9.5).

   Strip 8 is applied directly over strip 1 along the longitudinal axis of the arm (Fig. 9.6).

Lock strips   1. Re-apply anchor around the upper arm with 8-cm stretch tape without tension.
2. Using 3.75-cm tape, apply one half locking strip with tension over the shoulder from the base of the cheek and moving outwards to the acromioclavicular joint.

   The first strip starts on the posterior thoracic anchor and finishes just beyond the clavicle. The next strip starts on the clavicle and finishes on the anterior thoracic anchor. Continue in this manner, alternating posterior and anterior interlocking strips (Fig. 9.7).

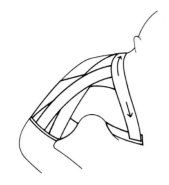

Figure 9.8

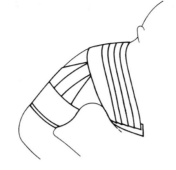

Figure 9.9

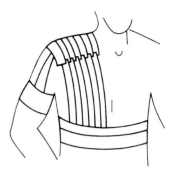

Figure 9.10

Alternative shoulder locking straps
O. Rouillon

Application
Apply strips of 4-cm tape directly over the shoulder with tension and attach to the anterior and posterior thoracic anchors. Lock with tape on the thoracic anchors (Figs 9.8 and 9.9).

Finish
Apply 10-cm cohesive bandage around the thorax a couple of times (Fig. 9.10).

Check function
Check efficiency of the tape job by lowering the elbow. Check tensions of the tape for stability of the acromioclavicular joint.

Tips
For sport such as rugby, apply padding over the tape job.

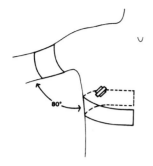

Figure 9.11

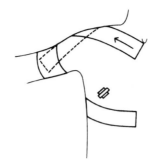

Figure 9.12

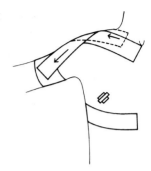

Figure 9.13

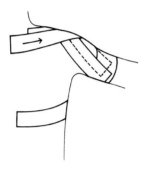

Figure 9.14

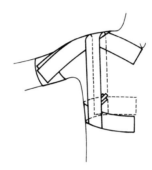

Figure 9.15

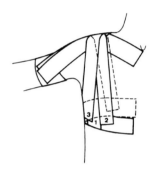

Figure 9.16

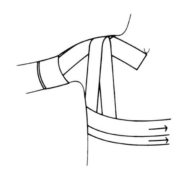

Figure 9.17

Acromioclavicular taping for sport using stretch tape

O. Rouillon

Indications
- Return to sport after acromioclavicular subluxation.
- Preventive for athletes with residual after-effects.
- For sprains where rigid tape is not necessary.

Function

Actively and passively to control the clavicle during sport.

Materials

Lubricant, three to four gauze squares, one to two rolls of 6-cm stretch tape, 10-cm cohesive bandage.

Position

Sitting with the arm abducted 80°.

Application

Protect the nipple with lubricant and pad. Protect the acromioclavicular joint with lubricant and pad.

Place an anchor of 6-cm stretch tape around the upper arm in the V of the deltoid without tension. Place a semicircular anchor around the thorax (Fig. 9.11).

Support strips

1. Using 6-cm stretch tape, start the first strip at the sternoclavicular joint and pull with moderate tension over the acromioclavicular joint to finish on the posterior aspect of the arm anchor (Fig. 9.12).
2. The second strip starts at the base of the neck and posteriorly crosses the acromioclavicular joint, finishing on the anterior aspect of the arm anchor (Fig. 9.13).
3. The third strip starts on the thoracic vertebra, crosses the acromioclavicular joint and finishes on the arm anchor anterior to strip 2 (Fig. 9.14).

Three more strips are applied (with 6-cm tape):

1. The first strip passes from the posterior thoracic anchor over the acromioclavicular joint, to finish on the anterior thoracic anchor in the sagittal plane (Fig. 9.15).
2. The second strip starts at a 30° angle to the first and crosses the first strip at the acromioclavicular joint.
3. The third strip is symmetrical to the second and crosses the previous two strips at the acromioclavicular joint (Fig. 9.16).

Anchors
(locking strips)

Using 6-cm stretch tape, repeat the initial anchors around the arm and thorax (Fig. 9.17).

To maintain the tape job in place, apply a 10-cm cohesive bandage a couple of times around the thorax.

Check function
- Test the active range of motion.
- Check if the tape job is supportive.

Chapter Ten

Elbow

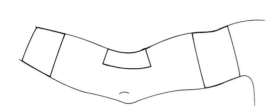

Figure 10.1

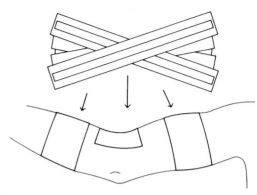

Figure 10.2

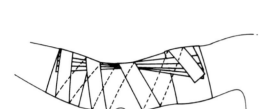

Figure 10.3

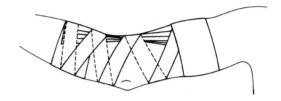

Figure 10.4

Elbow hyperextension taping procedure (Armstrong elbow)

C. Armstrong

Indications	Elbow pain: • Sprained inert tissue at the elbow • Strained elbow flexors
Function	1. To prevent further injury caused by hyperextension. 2. To prevent the elbow from fully extending or from reaching the point where pain begins.
Materials	Gauze squares, lubricant, adhesive spray, 5-/7.5-cm stretch tape, 3.75-cm tape, 10-cm cohesive bandage.
Position	The patient is standing with the arm held forwards, the palm up and the elbow flexed about 20° into the comfort zone.
Application	1. Shave the arm from the axilla to the distal-forearm. 2. Lubricate and apply gauze to the crease of the elbow. 3. Apply adhesive spray to the forearm and upper arm. 4. Apply an anchor strip (7.5-cm stretch tape) around the proximal end of the arm and following the contour of the biceps (Fig. 10.1). With 7.5-cm stretch tape, apply a second anchor around the mid-forearm following the upward sloping of the forearm musculature (Fig. 10.1). 5. Build and apply an hourglass fan of 3.75-cm tape with a 5-cm stretch tape centrepiece and border. The length of this hourglass fan will be enough to extend from the proximal edge of the proximal anchor to the distal edge of the distal anchor (Fig. 10.2). 6. Using 5-cm stretch tape begin a spiral of tape commencing at the proximal edge of the top anchor on the anteromedial aspect of the arm and moving anteriorly and laterally to cross the biceps, spiralling around the arm and securing the hourglass fan in place and coming around a second time to cross the crease of the elbow. Continue circling around the upper forearm to arrive at the distal anchor (Fig. 10.3). 7. Here the tape circles the forearm and continues back up the arm, continuing to spiral around this upper extremity, crossing the downwards spiral at right angles on the front of the arm and forming a symmetrical cross at the crease of the elbow. Continue up to cross the biceps and end at the proximal end of the upper anchor on the anterolateral aspect of the upper arm (Fig. 10.4). 8. Using 7.5-cm stretch tape, cover the proximal anchor. 9. Apply a 10-cm cohesive bandage over this tape job and leave it on for 10 minutes while the tape sets.
Check function	The patient should be limited from full extension or from reaching the point of pain when extending the elbow.
Contraindications	Circulation problems in the upper extremity.
Tips	• This procedure is best applied directly to the skin. • Have the patient hold the arm in 160° of extension or 20° short of where pain begins. • Use wider tape on larger people. • Have the patient flex the muscles when circling the limb with tape.

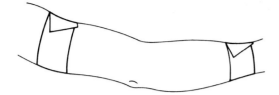

Figure 10.5

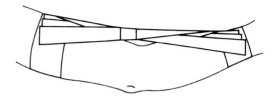

Figure 10.6

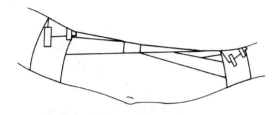

Figure 10.7a

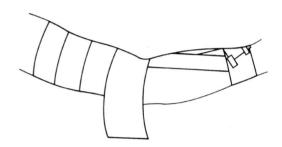

Figure 10.7b

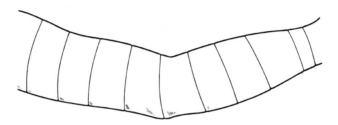

Figure 10.7c

Elbow hyperextension taping
K. Wright

Indication	Elbow sprains and strains.
Function	To provide support and stability to the elbow joint.
Materials	5-/7.5-cm stretch tape, 2.5-/3.75-cm adhesive tape.
Position	Elbow joint positioned in slight flexion.

Application

1. Apply two anchor strips of stretch tape. The proximal anchor will be positioned above the belly of the biceps muscle and the distal anchor will be positioned on the distal one-third of the forearm (Fig. 10.5).
2. Using 3.75-cm adhesive tape, construct a five- to seven-strip butterfly (hourglass) pattern that will extend from the proximal anchor to the distal anchor. Prior to application, place a strip of tape around the mid-portion of this support pattern (check rein, Fig. 10.6).
3. This butterfly pattern must be applied with the proper amount of tension to ensure that the elbow does not reach full extension.
4. A second series of anchor strips should be applied using stretch tape (Fig. 10.7a).
5. A final continuous closure strip is applied with 7.5-cm stretch tape. Begin on the proximal anchor and spiral the tape, overlapping one-half its width, and ending on the distal anchor (Fig. 10.7b).

Lock strips   Secure the stretch tape ends with adhesive tape strips (Fig. 10.7c).

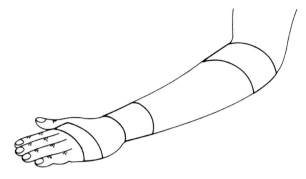

Figure 10.8

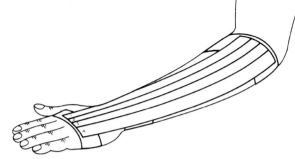

Figure 10.9

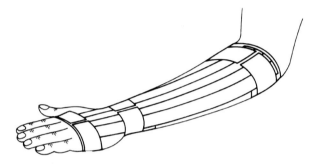

Figure 10.10

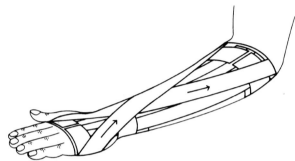

Figure 10.11

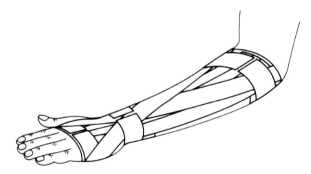

Figure 10.12

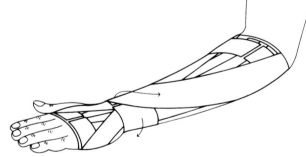

Figure 10.13

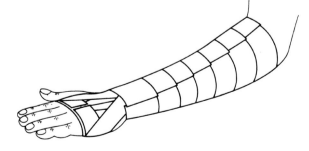

Figure 10.14

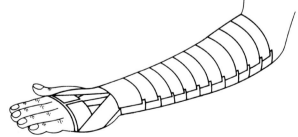

Figure 10.15

Tennis elbow–epicondylitis
O. Rouillon

Indication   Epicondylitis.

Function
- To limit wrist flexion.
- Radial and ulnar deviation.
- To limit tendon stretch.

Materials   Spray, pro-wrap, 3- and 6-cm stretch tape, 3.75-cm tape.

Position   The patient is sitting with the hand on the table, pronated.

Application   Spray the arm and hand, omitting the fingers. Apply pro-wrap from wrist to elbow.
1. Three anchors are used:
    (a) 6-cm stretch tape without tension proximally on forearm.
    (b) 6-cm tape around the wrist.
    (c) 3.75-cm adhesive tape; anchor it around the hand in a double semi-circular fashion without tension (Fig. 10.8).
2. Using 3.75-cm tape, apply four strips to the dorsum from the proximal anchor to the hand anchor, limiting flexion of fingers with the wrist in slight extension.
    (a) Strip 1 passes over the second metacarpal. The next three strips pass over the third, fourth and fifth metacarpals (Fig. 10.9).
    (b) The four strips are locked in place with three incomplete circles of tape placed over anchor points (Fig. 10.10).
3. Cut a 50-cm strip of 2.5-cm stretch tape. Place the palm of the hand on the centre of the strip behind the metacarpal heads. The radial strip passes over the dorsum of the wrist and is pulled with tension to attach to the proximal anchor on the lateral epicondyle. The ulnar strip is applied symmetrically, crossing the first at the wrist and attaching to proximal anchors (Fig. 10.11).
4. Lock these strips in place with 4-cm tape at the proximal and wrist anchors, in complete circular lock strips without tension (Fig. 10.12).
5. Using 6-cm stretch tape, start on the mid dorsal aspect of the wrist anchor. Wind around the ulnar to the palmar aspect over the radial head and pull with moderate tension obliquely up the arm to the epicondyle (Fig. 10.13).
6. Using 6-cm stretch tape, apply fill-in strips from the proximal to wrist anchors (Fig. 10.14).

Alternatively finish with fill-in strips–half-circles of 4-cm tape (Fig. 10.15) under and over.

Check function   Limitation of wrist flexion–also radial and ulnar deviation. Limits pronation.
In certain cases when the clinical examination shows that complete extension of the elbow causes pain, extension of the elbow must be limited by the wrappings.

Conclusion   This adhesive wrapping is an indispensable element of the therapy for epicondylitis.

Chapter Eleven

Hand and wrist

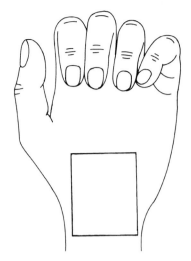

Figure 11.1

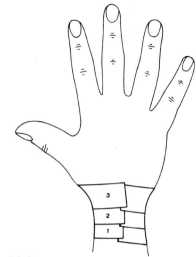

Figure 11.2

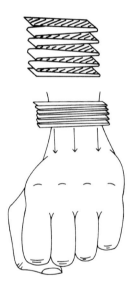

Figure 11.3

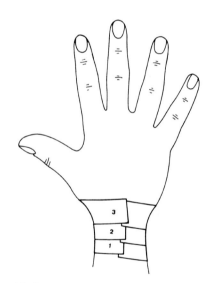

Figure 11.4

Prophylactic wrist taping

D. Reese

Indications	Prevention of injuries by wrist extension in sport, for example, in gymnastics, strength training and others.
Function	To reduce wrist extension by applying material over the dorsal aspect of the wrist, without causing the circulation and carpal tunnel problems often associated with supporting the wrist.
Materials	2.5-/3.75-cm tape, depending on the size of the wrist. A small piece of foam rubber, shaped to cover the palmar aspect of the wrist.
Position	Patient standing or sitting while making a fist.
Application	The patient should be clean, dry and shaved in the area to be taped. Start by having the patient actively make a fist. Place a spongy foam-rubber square on the palmar side of the wrist to protect the tendons (Fig. 11.1).
Anchors	Anchors 1, 2 and 3 should be placed starting approximately 5 cm proximal to the ulnar and radial styloid (Fig. 11.2). Apply the tape so that it conforms to the natural angle of the lower arm and hand junction. Overlap distally approximately one-third of the width of the first anchor. The bottom part of the last anchor should lie forward to the base of the second to fifth metacarpals. Check to see that the anchors do not constrict the range of motion.
Support	The support should cover the entire dorsal aspect of the wrist from the styloid processes to the base of the second to fifth metacarpals. The tape is taken back and forth over the area but never circular. The amount is dependent on the amount of support required. Five to six overlaps are common (Fig. 11.3).
Anchor lock	Anchors 1, 2 and 3 should be placed covering the first three (Fig. 11.4).
Check function	Is the wrist support adequate for the manoeuvre? If not, adjust by applying more material over the dorsal aspect of the wrist. Check action.
Contraindications	Circulation problems to the hand can occur if proper application is not followed. This taping is to be used only when the patient is active.
Tip	Best applied directly to the skin dorsally

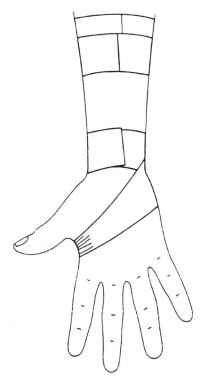

Figure 11.5

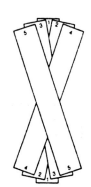

Figure 11.6

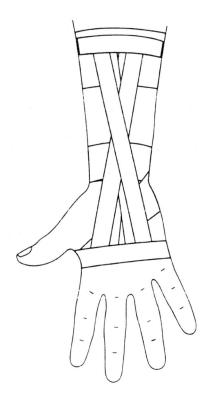

Figure 11.7

Wrist taping
R. Macdonald

Indication	Wrist hyperextension, hyperflexion injury.
Function	To support and limit range of motion.
Materials	Adhesive spray, underwrap, 3.75- and 2.5-cm tape.
Position	The hand is placed in the open position for anchors, facing operator.
Application	Spray the hand and wrist. When tacky, apply underwrap, making a hole with the thumb.
Anchors	1. Using 3.75-cm tape, apply a diagonal anchor across the hand and around the wrist, and two anchors around the mid-forearm below muscle bulk (Fig. 11.5). With the hand in a slightly flexed position, measure the distance between the proximal and hand anchors.
Check rein	2. Using 2.0-/2.5-cm tape, construct the check rein (fan) on the table (Fig. 11.6), overlapping each strip by half. 3. Apply the fan to anchors. Hold it in place manually and check the range of motion of the wrist joint, blocking full extension/flexion. Remember that the skin on the forearm is very mobile.
Lock strips	Apply strips across the ends of the fan to hold in place, then reapply the original anchors (Fig. 11.7). When applying tape: for hyperextension–slightly flex the wrist; for hyperflexion–slightly extend the wrist.
Check function	Is pronation/supination restricted? Can the patient hold the racquet/bat?
Tip	Wrap the hand and wrist with a waterproof cohesive bandage if the patient is going in water (swimmers or divers).

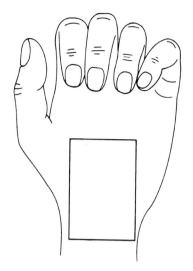

Figure 11.8

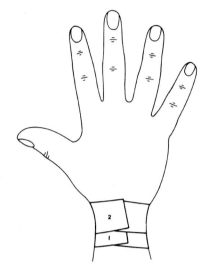

Figure 11.9

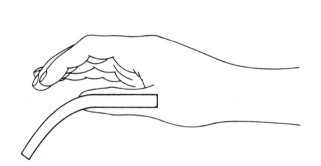

Figure 11.10

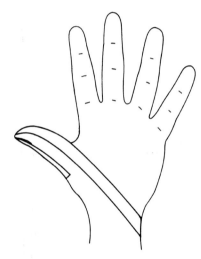

Figure 11.11

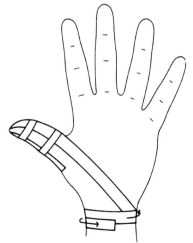

Figure 11.12

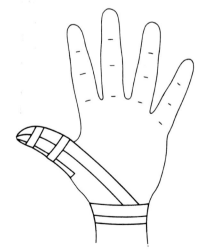

Figure 11.13

Prophylactic thumb taping
D. Reese

Indication	Prevention of injuries caused by hyperextension of the thumb in sports, for example, ice hockey, European handball, skiing, soccer goalkeepers, etc.
Function	To prevent hyperextension of the thumb and further damage to the volar ligament without inhibiting any other of the vital functions of the thumb. Its simplicity allows the athlete to regulate the tension at any time for better function.
Materials	2.5-/1.25-cm tape stripped (less than the width of the thumb). A small piece of foam rubber shaped to cover the palmar aspect of the wrist.
Position	The patient is standing or sitting.
Application	The hand should be clean, dry and shaved in the area to be taped. Start by having the patient actively make a fist. Place a spongy foam-rubber square on the palmar side of the wrist to protect the wrist tendons (Fig. 11.8).
Anchors	Anchors 1 and 2 should be placed starting approximately 5 cm proximal to the ulnar and radial styloid. Apply the tape so that it conforms to the natural angle of the lower arm and hand junction. Overlap distally approximately one-third of the width of the first anchor. Check to see that the anchors do not constrict the range of motion (Fig. 11.9).
Support	Place two strips 60 cm in length that are a little less than the width of the thumb on top of each other. Open the hand and start the support at the base of the first phalanx on the dorsal side of the hand. Pull the tape through the middle line of the thumb over the thumbnail and over the volar ligament towards the ulnar styloid on the palmar side of the hand (Figs 11.10 and 11.11). Wrap the rest of the support around the wrist (Fig. 11.12).
Lock strip	Lock a small strip around the second phalanx of the thumb as well as a couple of strips on top of each other over the base of the first phalanx (Fig. 11.13).
Check function	Allow the patient to decide the tension and restriction of the tape that will be used in the activity. Have on hand the equipment or ball for final adjustment.
Contraindication	Hypermobility in hyperextension of the thumb.
Tip	Inform the patient that adjustments may be made during the activity by pulling up the end of the tape and reapplying new tension around the wrist.

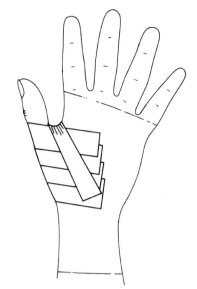

Figure 11.14

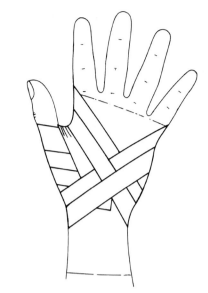

Figure 11.15

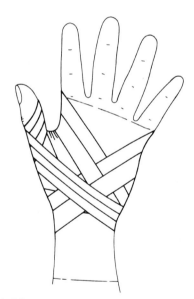

Figure 11.16

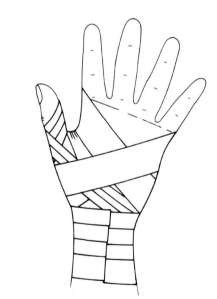

Figure 11.17

Boxer's hand wrap
J. O'Neill

Function	The function of this tape is to provide support and protect the hand. It is primarily used on offensive and defensive linemen in American football.
Materials	Adherent tape, underwrap, 5-cm light elastic wrap, 2.5-cm porous athletic tape, 3.75-cm porous athletic tape.
Position	The athlete should hold the wrist in a neutral position with the fingers spread as wide as possible.
Application	1. Tape adherent and underwrap should be placed from the base of the fingers to approximately 8–10 cm past the wrist.
	2. Apply 5-cm light elastic wrap, covering the hand and wrist completely.
	3. Apply three to four U-shaped strips (palmar to dorsal) using 2.5-cm tape, starting from the carpometacarpal joint of the thumb and proceeding upwards to the base of the metacarpophalangeal joint. Apply an anchor strip through the web to the thenar eminence (Fig. 11.14).
	4. Apply two to three basic figure-of-eights to the hand (Fig. 11.15).
	5. Follow this by two to three thumb spicas to the thumb (Fig. 11.16).
	6. Using 2.5-cm tape, wrap the hand, covering all open holes.
	7. Using 3.75-cm tape, apply three to four anchors to the wrist, each strip overlapping the preceding one by at least half its width (Fig. 11.17).
Check function	Make sure that the tape is not applied too tightly. This is an unusually large amount of tape, therefore we must watch for tightness around the thumb area. It is important that the athlete should have the hand and fingers spread during taping.

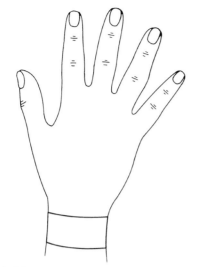

Figure 11.18

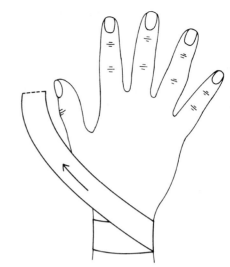

Figure 11.19

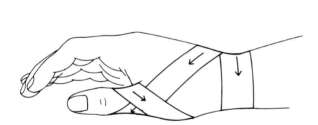

Figure 11.20

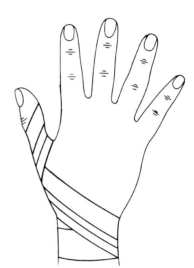

Figure 11.21

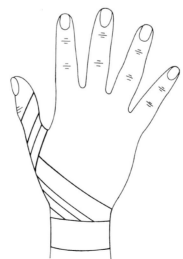

Figure 11.22

Thumb spica taping
K. Wright

Indication

Thumb sprain.

Function

To provide support and stability for the first metacarpophalangeal (thumb) joint.

Materials

2.5-cm adhesive tape.

Position

The hand is held in a palm-down position, with the thumb slightly flexed and the phalanges adducted.

Application

1. Apply an anchor strip of adhesive tape around the wrist (Fig. 11.18). Start at the ulnar condyle, cross the dorsal aspect of the distal forearm and encircle the wrist (Fig. 11.19).
2. Apply the first of three support strips for the first metacarpophalangeal joint. Starting at the ulnar condyle, cross the dorsum of the hand, cover the lateral joint line and circle the thumb. Proceed across the palmar aspect of the hand and finish at the ulnar condyle. This is commonly referred to as a thumb spica (Fig. 11.20).
3. Repeat this step twice. Overlap the tape by one-half its width, moving distally each time (Fig. 11.21).
4. Apply a final anchor strip around the wrist to help hold the procedure in place (Fig. 11.22).

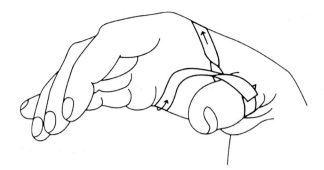

Figure 11.23a

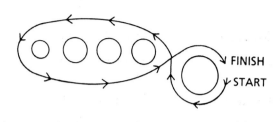

Figure 11.23b

Thumb, check rein figure-of-eight method

R. Macdonald

Indication	Thumb hyperextension (Fig. 11.23).
Function	To stabilize the joint and restrict extension and abduction of the thumb.
Materials	2.5-cm or 1.25-cm tape.
Position	The hand is held in a functional position. (Face the operator and shake hands.)
Application	Start on the dorsal aspect of the proximal aspect of the thumb. Draw tape around the thumb towards the palm, then through the web twisting the tape. Continue over the dorsal aspect of the hand, moulding the tape to the skin, then around and across the palmar surface to web moulding tape to the palm.
	Draw the thumb towards the palm into a functional position and attach the tape to the starting point (do not wind the end around the thumb).
	Apply this check rein over any thumb tape job.
	Note:
	● To control extension–apply tension towards the palmar surface.
	● To control abduction–apply tension towards the dorsal surface.
Tips	Use adhesive spray on the palm of the hand for better adhesion, and mould adhesive mass to the palm.
	Check circulation by pressing the thumb nail.

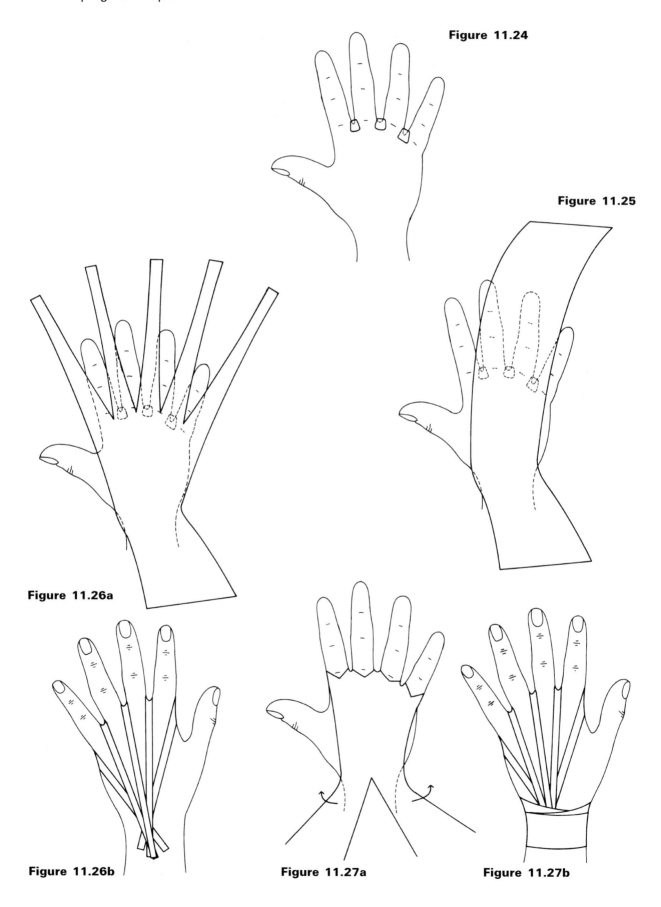

Figure 11.24

Figure 11.25

Figure 11.26a

Figure 11.26b

Figure 11.27a

Figure 11.27b

Palm protective taping (the Russell web)

C. Armstrong

Indication	Unconditioned/uncalloused palms in gymnastics.
Function	● To act as a layer of protection over the skin on the palm of the hand. ● To help the patient maintain a grip on gymnastic apparatus.
Materials	Adhesive spray, lubricant, 10-/7.5-cm stretch tape, 3.75-cm tape.
Position	The patient is standing with the arm held forwards and palm up.

Application

1. Shave the wrist.
2. Lubricate the web space between the fingers and apply gauze (Fig. 11.24).
3. Apply adhesive spray to the hand, including the wrist.
4. Using a length of 10-cm stretch tape that stretches to twice the length of the hand, attach the tape to the base of the hand so that the hand is in the middle of the length of tape (Fig. 11.25).
5. Starting at the finger-end of the tape, make four longitudinal cuts into the tape so that, when stretched, the tape strands fit between the fingers but the unsplit portion covers the palm (Fig. 11.26a).
6. Bring these taut strips up from the palmar aspect of the hand to go on the outside of the index finger on the one side and the little finger on the other. The middle strips come up into the web spaces between each of the fingers. These strips should run down the back of the hand, across the wrist, ending on the back of the distal forearm at the wrist (Fig. 11.26b).
7. Then, going to the wrist end of the length of tape, cut it down the middle, allowing the cut to correspond to the distal wrist crease. The two strips should be stretched and run around the wrist, anchoring the strands that come along the dorsum of the hand to the wrist (Fig. 11.27a).
8. Cover the wrist strips with 3.75-cm tape (Fig. 11.27b).

Check function

● The patient should be able to flex and extend the wrist without undue discomfort from the tape cutting into the web space between the fingers.
● The tape should be sufficiently taut not to allow any bunching.

Contraindications	None.
Tip	On a smaller hand, one might be well-advised to use 7.5-cm rather than 10-cm stretch tape.

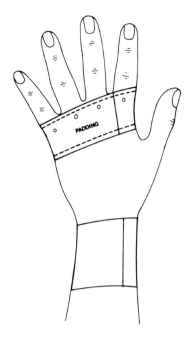

Figure 11.28

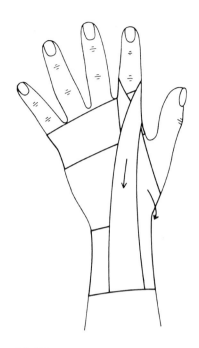

Figure 11.29

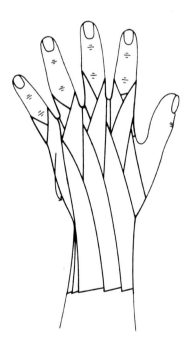

Figure 11.30

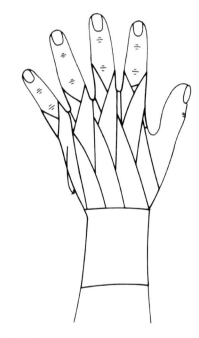

Figure 11.31

Protection of the metacarpophalangeal joints for boxers

R. Macdonald

Indication	To protect the metacarpophalangeal joints for boxers when training, and in combat sports.
Function	● To maintain the protective padding in place.
	● To leave the palm free for gripping in martial arts, judo, etc.
Materials	2.5 and 5-cm stretch tape, adhesive spray, padding/PPT/Poron or rubber.
Application	Spray the dorsum of the hand and wrist. Cut a protective pad to fit over the four metacarpophalangeal joints. Stick the pad in place and anchor it with 5-cm stretch tape. Apply 5-cm stretch tape anchor around the wrist (Fig. 11.28).
	Using 2.5-cm stretch tape, cut four strips long enough to encircle each finger and anchor on the proximal end of the wrist anchor.
	The centre of the first strip is placed around the index finger. Cross the two ends over the metacarpophalangeal joint. One winds over the metacarpal of the thumb to attach to the anterior aspect of the wrist anchor. The other end is attached to the wrist anchor, on the dorsum (Fig. 11.29).
	Repeat this on the middle and ring fingers. Finger 5 is the same as the index finger with one strip winding around to the palmar aspect of the wrist anchor (Fig. 11.30).
Lock strips	Reapply the wrist anchor and close off with the tape (Fig. 11.31).
	Note: The pad may be bevelled to overlay the web of the fingers or lubricated gauze pads may be applied between the fingers.
Check function	Can the athlete make a fist without discomfort? Is the pad in the right position for full protection?
Contraindications	None.
Tip	Apply adhesive spray directly to the pad. Let it get tacky before sticking it to the metacarpophalangeal joints. If secure, the anchor may not be necessary.

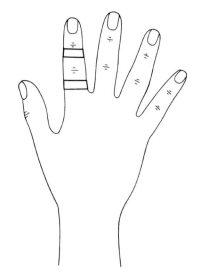

Figure 11.32

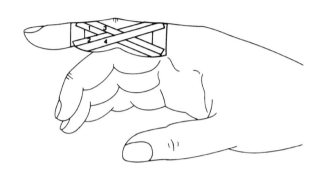

Figure 11.33

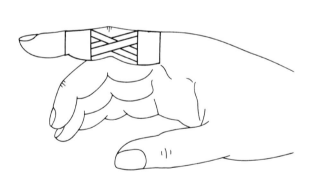

Figure 11.34

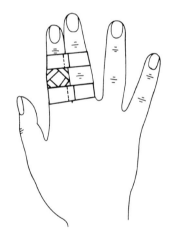

Figure 11.35

Sprained finger
J. O'Neil

Function	To help support the collateral ligaments of the fingers.
Materials	Tape adherent, 1.25-cm porous tape.
Position	The athlete's inured finger is extended in a relaxed position.
Application	This technique is similar to taping of collateral ligament sprain of a knee.

1. Apply tape adherent.
2. Apply a 1.25-cm anchor strip around the middle and proximal phalanx (Fig. 11.32).
3. Eight strips of 1.25-cm tape approximately 5–8 cm long are precut and then applied as indicated in Figure 11.33.
4. Place a 2.5-cm strip to cover tape around the middle and proximal phalanx (Fig. 11.34).
5. Finally, 'buddy tape' the injured finger to the adjacent finger to aid in support (Fig. 11.35).

Check function	Be watchful of overtightness of the tape.
Tip	When taping fingers, place in about 15° of flexion. This will allow the athlete to feel more comfortable.

Chapter Twelve

Stretch tape – many uses

R. Macdonald

One is sometimes in a position when there is a minimum supply of tape available for use. One strip of tape may be adapted for many uses and in many cases, lends itself to self-application. The following are some ideas for using a length of stretch tape with its ends cut or torn into four tails. The adhesive mass on the uncut centre portion may be covered with another piece–sticky sides together–or reinforced with a piece of rigid tape for more strength. The application of talcum powder to the adhesive side eliminates the sticky mass from the tape.

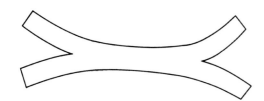

Figure 12.1   7.5/10-cm stretch tape

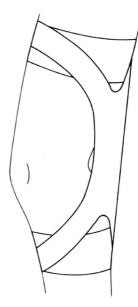

Figure 12.2   Tape used to block full knee extension

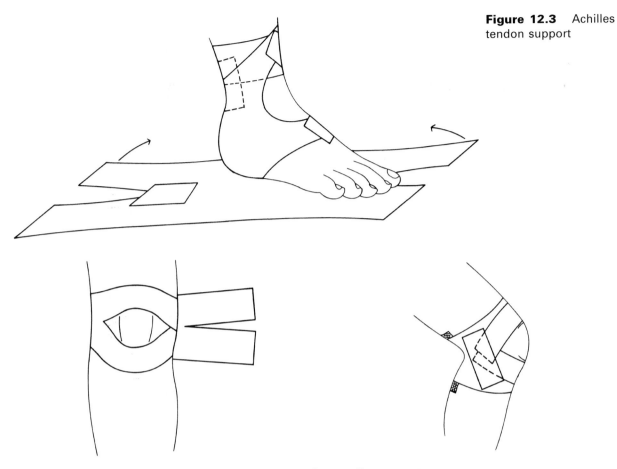

Figure 12.3 Achilles tendon support

Figure 12.4 (a and b) 7.5/10-cm stretch tape used for patellar support

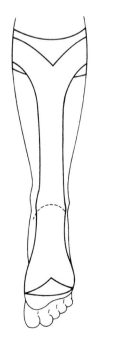

Figure 12.5 Achilles tendon support

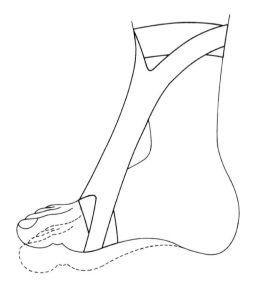

Figure 12.6 Tape used to support dorsiflexors (dropped foot)

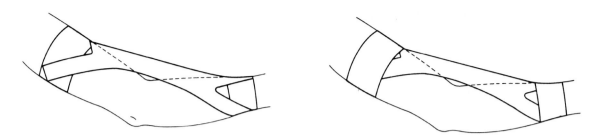

Figure 12.7 (a and b) To block full extension of the elbow

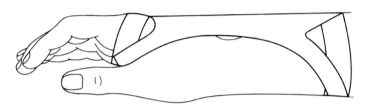

Figure 12.8 Tape used to support extensor tendons (dropped wrist)

Chapter Thirteen

Spicas

R. Macdonald

The spica or figure-of-eight bandage is very useful for a variety of conditions and can often be self-applied. In some situations, the spica is more appropriate than tape and is often used as a first-aid measure to protect the injured structure, to restrict range of motion and to minimize swelling and bleeding. Elastic or stretch tape or any type of non-adhesive bandage may be used. If the support is to be removed for the application of cold or heat or therapeutic exercise, then a bandage is more appropriate as it may be used many times and is less costly. The spica must be applied firmly but not too tightly, each strip overlapping the previous one by half. A cold, wet spica is ideal for an acute injury. After application, check circulation and neural transmission.

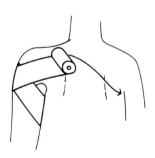

a

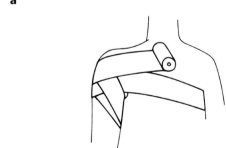

b

Figure 13.1   (a) and (b) Shoulder spica

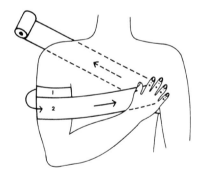

a

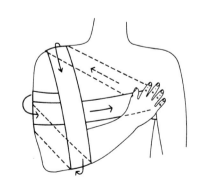

b

Figure 13.2   (a) and (b) Bandage to support a dislocation of the acromioclavicular and/or a shoulder joint

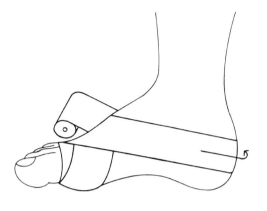

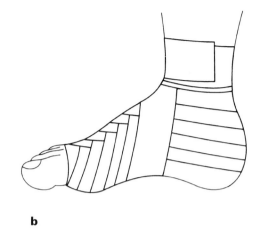

a

b

Figure 13.3 (a) and (b) Ankle and foot spica

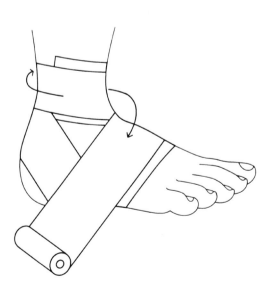

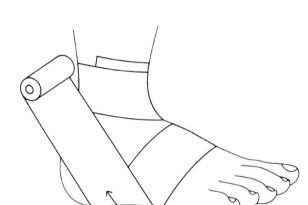

a

b

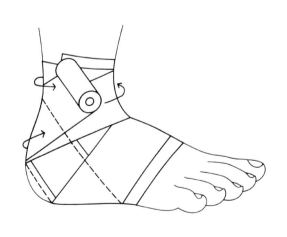

c

d

Figure 13.4 (a–d) Ankle wrap

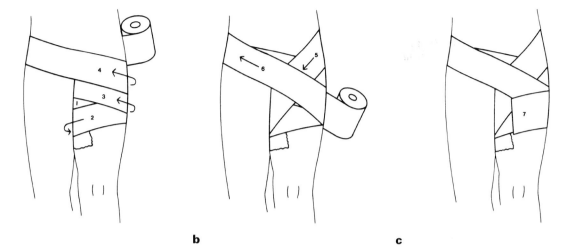

a   **b**   **c**

Figure 13.5   (a–c) Elastic groin support

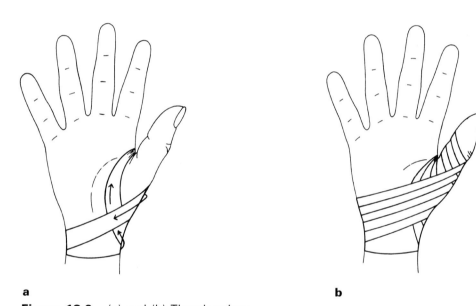

a   **b**

Figure 13.6   (a) and (b) Thumb spicas

Chapter Fourteen

Basic first aid

C. Stretton

Aims

- To preserve life
- To prevent the condition deteriorating
- To promote recovery

Develop a simple routine: this will help you to keep a clear head and give care in a logical order.

Go quickly but calmly to the scene of the incident. Remember to take your first-aid kit with you.

Assess

- Evaluate what has happened.
- Estimate who and how many are injured.
- Look carefully; don't jump to hasty conclusions.

Make safe

- Don't take risks.
- Ensure the safety of the casualty and yourself–this may mean stopping all activities in the area (Fig. 14.1).

Give help

Urgent treatment

A   Maintain a clear *airway*.
B   If the casualty is no longer *breathing*, give mouth-to-mouth ventilation.

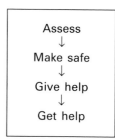

Figure 14.1 Help routine. © Order of St. John 1993. All rights reserved

C   If the casualty's *circulation* has stopped, apply external cardiac compressions. *Control* severe bleeding.

Important treatment

- Cover wounds.
- Immobilize and support fractures.
- Place the casualty in the correct and most comfortable position.

Helpful treatment

- Give reassurance and sympathy.
- Handle the casualty gently to reduce pain and minimize further damage.
- Protect the casualty from the cold and damp.

Get help

This may involve:
- Obtaining help from a colleague or bystander

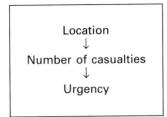

Figure 14.2 To obtain an ambulance, give this information. © Order of St. John 1993. All rights reserved

- Informing a parent
- Referral to the casualty's own doctor
- Obtaining an ambulance (Fig. 14.2)

Record

- Details of all incidents treated
- Details of care given
- Time scale

If the casualty appears unconscious, follow the ABC of resuscitation (see below).

Tip: Remember, the noisiest casualty is rarely the most seriously injured.

ABC of resuscitation

Act quickly

Check the response: gently shake the casualty's shoulders and shout 'wake up'. If there is no response:

A: Clear the airway

Turn the casualty's head to one side. Using two fingers, carefully remove any obvious debris from inside the mouth. Leave well-fitting dentures in place.

Open the airway

Lift the chin using the index and middle fingers of one hand. Press the forehead backwards using the heel of the other hand (Fig. 14.3).

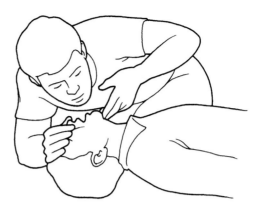

Figure 14.3 Open the airway. © Order of St. John 1993. All rights reserved

B: Check the breathing

- Look for chest movement.
- Listen and feel for exhaled air.

If the casualty is breathing, turn him or her into the recovery position. Obtain help.

If casualty is not breathing: *send for medical help immediately.* Start artificial ventilation.

Artificial ventilation

- Pinch the casualty's nose with your thumb and forefinger.
- Take a deep breath.
- Seal your lips around the casualty's lips (Fig. 14.4a).
- Blow slowly into the casualty's mouth–watch the chest rise and fall (Fig. 14.4b).
- Give a second inflation.

C: Check the carotid pulse

If present:

- Continue inflations at a rate of 10 per minute.
- Check the carotid pulse after every 10 breaths (Fig. 14.5).
- When normal breathing resumes, turn the casualty into the recovery position.

If not present:

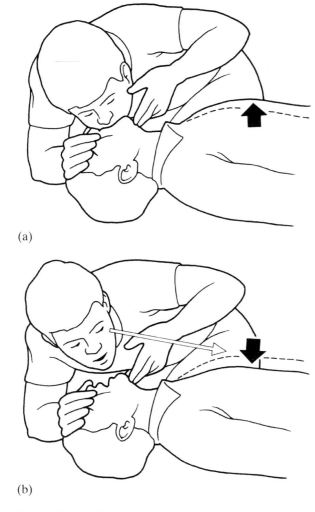

(a)

(b)

Figure 14.4 Artificial ventilation. © Order of St. John 1993. All rights reserved

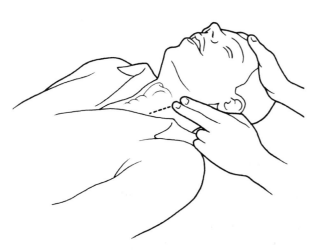

Figure 14.5 Checking the carotid pulse. © Order of St. John 1993. All rights reserved

Start chest compressions

- Place the heel of your hand two fingers-breadth above the junction of the ribcage and the sternum. Place the other hand on top and interlock the fingers.
- Keeping your arms straight, lean over the casualty, depress the sternum 4–5 cm. Release pressure. Repeat the compressions 14 times at a rate of approximately 80 times per minute (Fig. 14.6).

Give two mouth-to-mouth ventilations followed by 15 chest compressions.

Do not break the sequence to check the pulse unless there are signs of returning circulation.

Once the heart beat resumes, continue inflating the casualty at a rate of 10 breaths per minute.

When two first-aiders are present, one summons help while the other starts resuscitation immediately. Two first-aiders working together maintain one inflation followed by five chest compressions.

Ensure the chest rises but do not wait for the chest to fall between compressions.

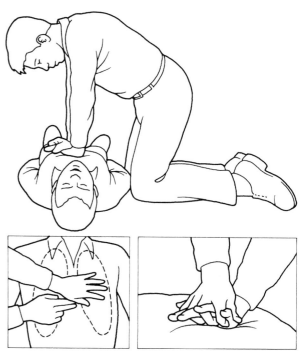

Figure 14.6 Chest compression. © Order of St. John 1993. All rights reserved

Cardiopulmonary resuscitation (CPR)

One first-aider

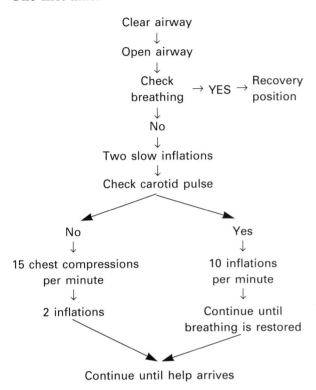

Clear airway
↓
Open airway
↓
Check breathing → YES → Recovery position
↓
No
↓
Two slow inflations
↓
Check carotid pulse

No ← ↓ → Yes

No
↓
15 chest compressions per minute
↓
2 inflations

Yes
↓
10 inflations per minute
↓
Continue until breathing is restored

Continue until help arrives

Figure 14.7

Two first-aiders

Give cardiopulmonary resuscitation at a rate of one inflation followed by five compressions (Fig. 14.7).

Choking

Conscious adults

- Encourage coughing.
- Bend the casualty forward, with the head lower than the lungs.
- Slap him or her firmly between the shoulder blades (Fig. 14.8a).
- Repeat up to five times.
- Check the mouth and hook out the obstruction.

If unsuccessful, apply *abdominal thrust:*

- Stand or kneel behind the casualty.

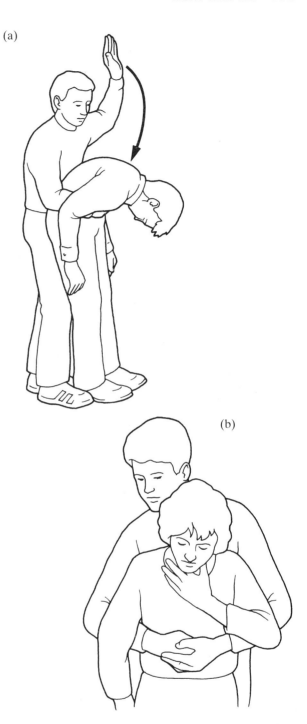

(a)

(b)

Figure 14.8 (a and b) Treatment of choking in a conscious adult. © Order of St. John 1993. All rights reserved

- Place the clenched-fist thumb inwards in the centre of the abdomen between the navel and sternum.
- Grasp the fist with the other hand (Fig. 14.8b).

- Pull both hands towards you with a quick upward and inward thrust.
- Repeat up to four times.
- Check the mouth again.

If necessary, repeat backslaps and abdominal thrusts.

Unconscious adults

- Turn the casualty on to his or her side facing you, with the head extended.
- Slap firmly between the shoulder blades, up to five times (Fig. 14.9a).
- Check the mouth.

If the obstruction is not cleared:

- Place the casualty on his or her back.
- Open the airway.
- Kneel astride or alongside the casualty's thighs.
- Place the heel of the hand in the centre of the upper abdomen; cover it with the other hand (Fig. 14.9b).
- Keep the arms straight and give a quick inward and upward thrust.
- Repeat up to four times.

Repeat the previous stages until they are effective.

Be prepared to resuscitate.

Tip: Do not practise the abdominal thrust on people: it may cause injury.

Suspected heart attack

Clues

- Severe vice-like pain in the chest
- The patient may complain of severe indigestion
- Breathlessness
- Sudden faintness and giddiness
- Ashen skin, cyanosis of lips and extremities
- Profuse sweating
- Rapid pulse, becoming weaker and irregular

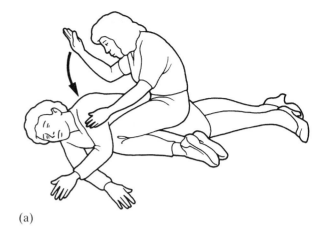

(a)

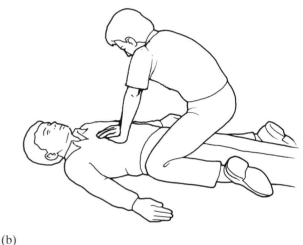

(b)

Figure 14.9 (a and b) Treatment of choking in an unconscious adult. © Order of St. John 1993. All rights reserved

Aims

- To minimize the work of the heart
- To obtain urgent medical aid
- To arrange transfer to hospital

Care

- Do not move the casualty unnecessarily.
- Help the casualty into the most comfortable position–half-sitting, with knees bent.
- Obtain medical aid: state a suspected heart attack.
- Monitor breathing and pulse rate constantly.
- Be prepared to resuscitate.

General care of the unconscious casualty

Aims

- Ensure an open airway.
- Monitor changes in casualty's condition.
- Seek medical aid.
- Protect the patient's interests.

Rapid assessment

- Alert
- Response to voice
- Response to pain
- No response

Care

- Maintain airway.
- Monitor breathing.
- Control serious bleeding.
- Establish levels of responsiveness.
- Support fractures.
- Place the patient in the recovery position.
- Cover him or her with a blanket.
- Check and record responses every 10 minutes.
- Transfer to hospital.

Do not

- Give anything by mouth.
- Leave the casualty unattended.
- Move the casualty unnecessarily.

Tip: Check for Medi-Alert bracelets, warning talisman or cards. Pass on your notes to hospital.

Levels of response

Eyes open

- Spontaneously
- To speech
- To pain
- No response

Movement

- Obeys commands
- Responds to painful stimuli
- No response

Speech

- Normal
- Confused
- Incomprehensible
- No response

Record the pulse and respiration rate.
Note the time and level of response every 10 minutes.

Recovery position

All unconscious casualties who are breathing and whose heart is beating must be turned into the recovery position to prevent the tongue from obstructing the airway and to prevent the inhalation of saliva and regurgitated stomach contents.

Method

- Remove spectacles.
- Open the airway.
- Straighten the patient's legs.
- Place the casualty's nearest arm at right angles, palm uppermost.
- Bring the casualty's far arm across the chest, placing the back of the hand against the casualty's cheek and hold.
- With your other hand, grasp the far thigh behind the knee and pull the knee up.

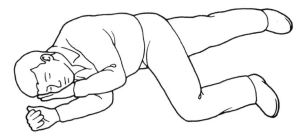

Figure 14.10 Recovery position. © Order of St. John 1993. All rights reserved

- Still holding the casualty's hand against the cheek, hold the flexed thigh and pull the casualty on to his or her side, towards you (Fig. 14.10).
- Confirm the airway is open.
- Adjust the casualty's top leg to ensure hip and knee are flexed at right angles.
- Monitor breathing and pulse rate.

Head injuries

Head injuries may result in damage to or disturbance of the brain and are potentially serious. Always seek medical advice. Any blow severe enough to cause a wound may have caused damage to the skull and brain.

Concussion

This is temporary disturbance of the brain caused by:
- A blow to the head
- A fall from a height on to feet
- A blow to the chin

Clues

- Brief or partial loss of consciousness
- Pale face
- Cold and clammy skin
- Rapid and weak pulse
- Shallow breathing

On recovery the patient:
- May feel sick and vomit
- May have loss of memory of events just before or after the accident

Care

- In mild cases, place the casualty in the care of a responsible person.
- Stress the need to seek medical advice.
- If the patient is unconscious, carry out the treatment detailed in the section on general care of the unconscious above.
- Watch for signs and symptoms of compression developing.

Do not allow casualty to play on without seeking medical approval.

Compression

A serious condition, requiring urgent treatment, may develop following concussion or up to 48 hours post injury.

Clues

- Severe headache
- Breathing becomes noisy
- Flushed face, raised temperature
- Pulse slow but strong
- Unequal pupils
- Weakness or paralysis on one side of the body
- Deterioration in levels of response

Care

- General care of unconscious casualty
- Urgent removal to hospital

Fainting

Aim

- To improve blood supply to the brain and care whilst the patient is unconscious.

Impending faint

Care

- Lay or sit the casualty down with his or her head between the knees.
- Loosen tight clothing.
- Reassure and support.

Actual faint

Clues

- Unconscious
- Pale face

- Cold and clammy skin
- Shallow breathing
- Weak and slow pulse, which gradually increases in rate

Care

- Maintain the airway.
- Raise the lower limbs.
- Loosen tight clothing.
- Ensure a supply of fresh air.
- On recovery, gradually allow the casualty to sit up.
- Sips of water may be given–but no alcohol.

If unconsciousness persists, follow routine care of the unconscious casualty.

Care of the epileptic casualty

Aims

- Protection of the casualty from injury
- Care whilst unconscious
- Care on recovery

Care

- Ease the casualty's fall.
- Clear space around.
- Loosen clothing at the neck.
- Support the casualty's head.
- Place the patient in the recovery position when the fit ceases.
- Stay with the casualty until recovery is complete.
- Advise the casualty to contact his or her own doctor.

Transfer the casualty to hospital if he or she is unconscious for more than 10 minutes or fits recur.

Tip: Do not forcibly restrain the casualty or put anything into his or her mouth.

Shock

Shock is always present when injuries occur, especially when severe bleeding or severe pain is present. It varies from faintness to complete collapse.

Aims

- To maintain adequate blood supply to vital centres
- To obtain medical aid as necessary

Care

- Reassure and comfort.
- Lay the casualty down with his or her head low and turned to one side.
- Raise the patient's legs.
- Prevent heat loss.
- Examine and treat cause of shock.
- Monitor breathing.
- If the casualty becomes unconscious, turn him or her into the recovery position.
- Obtain help.

Do not

- Remove clothes unnecessarily.
- Give fluids by mouth.
- Allow the casualty to smoke.

Tip: When the face is pale, lift the tail.

Control of bleeding

Aims

- To prevent blood loss
- To limit infection to the casualty and to yourself
- To prevent shock

Immediate care

- Expose the wound.
- Apply direct pressure over a sterile dressing or press the edges together with your fingers.
- Lay the casualty down.
- Elevate and support the limb.
- Cover the wound with a sterile dressing; secure it firmly (Fig. 14.11a).

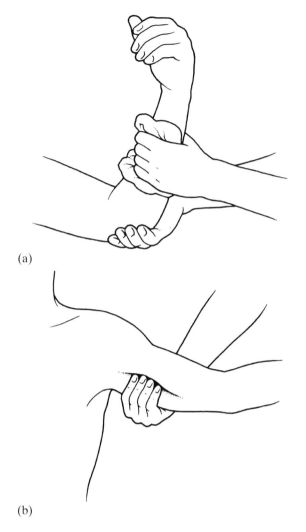

(a)

(b)

Figure 14.11 Control of bleeding. (a) Direct pressure; (b) indirect pressure. © Order of St. John 1993. All rights reserved

- Reassure the patient.
- Obtain medical aid.

Further care

- Check the dressing frequently for signs of further bleeding.
- If bleeding continues, place another dressing on top of the first and secure firmly. Do *not* remove original dressing.

If bleeding still continues, apply pressure to the main artery supplying the limb (Fig. 14.11b). Maintain pressure for periods of 10 minutes only.
Do not apply a tourniquet.

Foreign bodies

If they are small and superficial, remove them. Do not attempt to remove larger embedded objects.

Build dressings up around the wound higher than the object, then bandage. Immobilize the limb.

Tip: Wear disposable gloves when giving care. Wash the hands well before and after removing gloves. Cover personal wounds.

Puncture wounds

These have a small entry, causing a deep wound. The risk of infection is high as germs and dirt may have been carried deep into the tissues.

Care

- Do not wash.
- Cover with a sterile dressing.
- Seek medical advice.

Tip: The risk of tetanus infection is greater in dirty wounds, especially if they are contaminated by soil, grit or gravel. Casualties who have not had anti-tetanus protection or whose last injection was more than 10 years ago must be told to seek medical advice.

Bleeding from the nose

Care

- Sit the casualty down, with the head well forward.
- Pinch the soft part of the nose firmly for 10 minutes.
- Repeat as necessary.

Do not

- Plug the nose.
- Blow the nose.
- Continue vigorous exercise.

If bleeding persists, seek medical advice.

Bleeding from the mouth, tongue and lips

Aims

- To safeguard breathing
- To control bleeding

Care

- Sit the casualty down.
- Keep the casualty's head forward, inclined to the injured side.
- Using a clean handkerchief or dressing, compress the wound between finger and thumb.
- Instruct the casualty to spit out any blood.
- If bleeding persists, seek medical advice.

Knocked-out teeth

Care

- Replace the tooth in the socket, the correct way around.
- Do not attempt to clean the tooth.
- Press it firmly into position.
- Have the patient see a dentist.

Tip: If the tooth cannot be replaced, place it in a cup of milk and seek dental advice.

General wound care

Minor wounds

Aims

- To prevent infection
- To promote healing

Care

- If possible, wash your hands before giving treatment.
- If the wound is dirty, rinse it under a running tap.
- Dry it gently.
- If bleeding persists, apply direct pressure.
- Cover it with an adhesive dressing.

A larger wound will need a gauze dressing.

Abrasions

These wounds are extremely painful and have a high risk of infection.

Care

- Rinse the abrasion under a cold running tap to remove small pieces of grit.
- Gentle wiping with a piece of gauze may also help to remove debris.
- Cover the wound with a non-adherent dressing.
- Seek medical advice.

Treatment of suspected fractures

Aims

- To prevent movement at site of injury
- To arrange removal to hospital

Clues

- Pain and tenderness
- Swelling
- Loss of power
- Deformity

Compare with the uninjured limb.

Care

- Tell the casualty to keep still.
- Treat at the scene of the accident.
- Steady and support the injured limb by hand until it is immobilized.
- Treat shock.
- Elevate the limb if possible.

Upper limbs

- Using a sling, support the arm against the trunk.
- Remove any rings before swelling occurs.

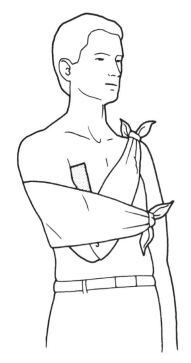

Figure 14.12 Treatment of a fractured collar bone. ©
Order of St. John 1993. All rights reserved

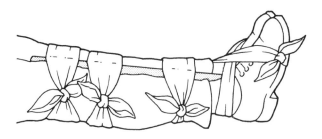

Figure 14.13 Treatment of a fractured lower limb. ©
Order of St. John 1993. All rights reserved

Collar bone

Clues

- Pain and tenderness at fracture site
- Reluctance to move arm on injured side
- The casualty supports the arm at the elbow
  and tilts the head to the injured side

Care

- Place the arm on the injured side across the
  chest, with the fingertips to the opposite
  shoulder.

- Support it in an elevation sling.
- Secure the arm to the chest (Fig. 14.12).
- Take or send the patient to hospital.

Lower limbs

- Steady and support the injured part in the
  most comfortable position until an
  ambulance arrives.
- If removal is delayed, secure the sound leg
  to the injured one by bandaging above and
  below the fracture, feet and knees.
  Remember to pad well (Fig. 14.13).

**Open fracture (when there is a wound leading
down to the fracture or bone protrudes)**

- Steady and support, as before.
- Cover the wound with a large sterile gauze
  dressing, pad well, building the dressing
  higher than the protruding bone.
- Secure firmly to control any bleeding.
- Immobilize.

Tip: Do not give the casualty anything to eat or
drink.

Dislocations

Clues

- Severe pain over joint
- Fixed joint
- Deformity
- Swelling

Do not attempt to replace bones to their
normal position.

Care

- Steady and support the limb in the most
  comfortable position.
- Immobilize.
- Transfer the casualty to hospital.

Soft tissue damage

Aim

- To reduce pain and swelling

Care

R: Rest the injured part,
I: Apply ice or cold compress,
C: Compress injury, pad well, bandage firmly,
E: Elevate limb.

First aid for long-distance runners

Hypothermia

This may occur in:
- Poorly clad runners on a cold, wet day
- Slow-moving runners who started too fast and become exhausted

Clues

- Feels cold
- Looks cyanosed
- Muscular cramps
- Confused

Care

- Remove wet clothing.
- Dry well.
- Make a warm environment.
- Provide dry clothes and a warm blanket.
- Give a warm, sweet drink.
- Record the rectal temperature, if possible. If it is less than 36°C and not improving, seek medical aid.

Hyperthermia

This is common on hot, humid days.

Clues

- Skin may be cool and dry, or the patient may be sweating profusely with severe generalized cramps.
- Rectal temperature is over 40°C.

Care

- Start tepid sponging.
- Fan.
- Give cool fluids.
- If there is no fall in temperature, transfer the patient to hospital urgently.

Hypovolaemic collapse

Long-distance runners may lose large quantities of fluid, causing hypotension. They may collapse 20–30 minutes after they stop running.

Clues

- May faint
- Pulse weak and imperceptible at wrist–check the carotid
- Feels dizzy
- May vomit

Care

- The casualty responds well to rest.
- Raise the patient's legs for 30 minutes at least.
- Give oral fluids in small quantities and frequently.
- If vomiting or diarrhoea persists, seek medical aid.

Tip: When replacing fluid loss orally, plain water is tolerated the best.

Application of bandages and dressings

Basic rules

- Sit or lay the casualty down.
- Sit or stand in front of the part to be bandaged.
- Support the injured part.
- Do not tie over bony areas.
- Tie knots to the front on the uninjured side.
- Always place padding between ankles and knees before tying together.

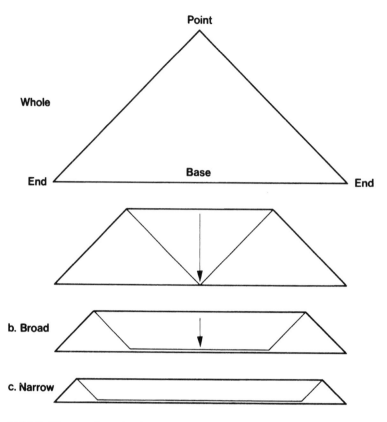

Figure 14.14 Folding a triangular bandage. © Order of St. John 1993. All rights reserved

- If the casualty is lying down, use natural hollows (back, knees, ankles) to pass bandages under the body. Gently ease into position.

When tying always use a *reef knot*, which lies flat, doesn't slip and is easy to untie.
Always check the circulation regularly after tying bandages.

Triangular bandages (Fig. 14.14)

These may be used open as a sling, or folded:
- to maintain pressure
- to prevent swelling
- to provide support
- to restrict movement

Arm sling

This is used for injuries to upper limbs and some chest injuries.

It is only effective if the casualty sits or stands.
Note: The casualty's hand should be slightly higher than the elbow. The finger nails should be exposed (Fig. 14.15).

Elevation sling (Fig. 14.16)

- Supports the hand and forearm in a well-raised position
- Helps to control bleeding
- Helps to reduce swelling

Improvization

- If an anorak or jacket is worn, turn up the lower edge over the injured arm and pin it firmly to the body of the jacket.
- A scarf, tights or a belt may also be used.

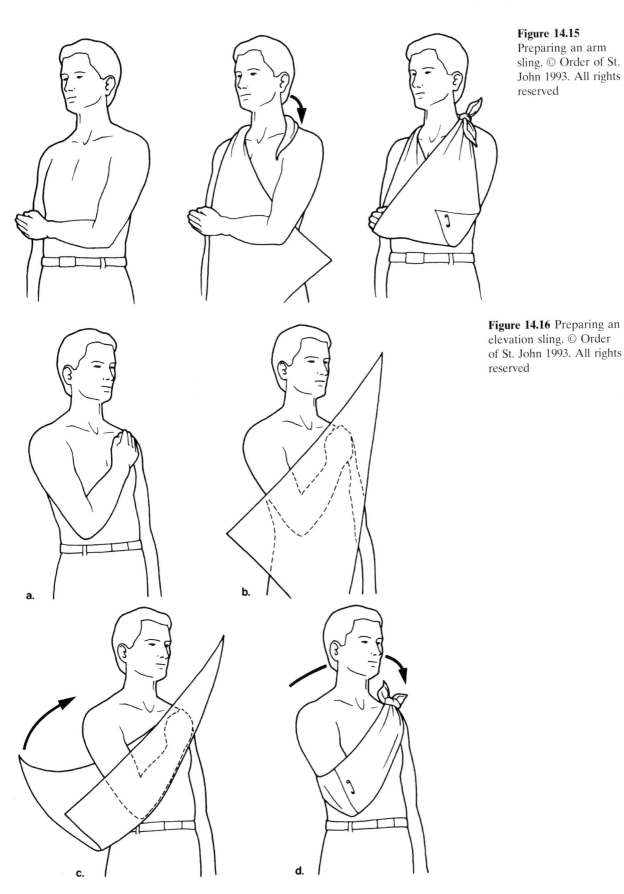

Figure 14.15
Preparing an arm
sling. © Order of St.
John 1993. All rights
reserved

Figure 14.16 Preparing an
elevation sling. © Order
of St. John 1993. All rights
reserved

a.

b.

c.

d.

Basic first-aid kit

The container should be waterproof and durable.

Contents

- Adhesive dressings, assorted sizes, individually wrapped
- Sterile unmedicated emergency dressings, medium and large sizes
- Sterile eye pads
- Sterile gauze squares
- Triangular bandages
- Non-adherent dressings
- Cotton wool
- Crêpe bandages
- Adhesive tape
- Scissors
- Safety pins
- Polythene bags (small)
- Tissues
- Note paper and pencil
- Disposable gloves

Quantities are determined by individual needs.

Tip: Kit must be easy to recognize and easy to carry.

Whilst these notes are valuable, a first-aid course is essential.

Glossary

Abduction movement	Away from the midline of the body
Achilles tendon	Tendon behind heel
Adduction movement	Towards the midline of the body
Adhesive mass	Sticky backing on tape
Anterior	Front
Anterior cruciate	Ligament within the knee joint
Assess	Evaluate
Biceps	Muscle on front of upper arm
Calcaneum	Heel bone
Check rein	Reinforced tape to prevent movement
Cohesive bandage	Rubberized, sticks to itself and not to the skin
Condyle	Bony end of thigh bone
Contract	Tense
Contusion	Bruise
Digit	Finger/toe
Distal	Area away from centre of body or furthest attachment
Dorsal	Back (e.g. of hand)
Extension	To straighten
Extensor tendons	On front of ankle joint
Femur	Thigh bone
Flexion	To bend
Friction	Rubbing
Hamstring	Muscle at back of thigh
Hyperextend	To extend beyond the normal
Hypoallergenic	Will not cause reaction on sensitive skin
Inferior	Below
Kinesiology	Study of motion of human body
Lateral	Side away from the body–outside
Ligaments	Taut bands of tissue which bind bones together
Longitudinal arch	From heel to toes on under surface of foot
Malleolus	Ankle bone
Medial	Side closest to the body–inside
Palmar	Front (e.g. of hand)
Patella	Knee cap
Peritendinitis	Inflammation of the Achilles paratenon

Plantar fascia	Tough bands of tissue on sole of foot
Plantar fasciitis	Inflammation at origin of plantar fascia (near heel)
Plantarflex	Toes and foot pointed towards floor
Plinth	Couch or bed
Popliteal fossa	Space behind knee
Posterior	Behind
Prone	Lying face-down
Pronate	Turn palm-down
Pronated feet	Flat feet
Proprioception	Awareness of body position, perception of movement and change of direction
Proximal	Close to centre of body or nearest attachment
Quadriceps	Muscles at front of thigh
Rehabilitate	To treat and restore to normal health
Superior	Above
Supinate	Turn palm up
Supine	Lying on the back
Thenar eminence	Muscular area of thumb on palm of hand
Tibia	Shin bone
Tibial tubercle	Attachment of patellartendon
Transverse arch	From medial to lateral

Index

516 LBIC
8/4/94 Y10-2 37 CLB

77 310PT 5538
BR
09/99 01-625-00 GBC